Pseudocereals

Edited by Viduranga Y. Waisundara

Published in London, United Kingdom

Pseudocereals
http://dx.doi.org/10.5772/intechopen.98152
Edited by Viduranga Y. Waisundara

Contributors
Noorazwani Zainol, Harisun Yaakob, Dayang Norulfairuz Abang Zaidel, Nor Hasmaliana Abdul Manas, Nurul Elia Aqila Abu Rahim, Norsuhada Abdul Karim, Luis Olivera, Perla Paredes, Neyma Perez, Luis Chong, Alejandro Marzano, Ivan Best, Svetlana Motyleva, Murat Gins, Valentina Gins, Nikolay Tetyannikov, Ivan Kulikov, Ludmila Kabashnikova, Daria Panischeva, Maria Mertvischeva, Irina Domanskaya, Padamnabhi Nagar, Riya Engineer, Krishna Rajput, Viduranga Y. Waisundara, Asel C. Weerasekara, Kanchana Priyadarshani Samarasinghe, Tatiana Bojňanská, Alena Vollmannová, Janette Musilová, Judita Lidiková, Asli Can Karaca, Upasana, Latika Yadav, Amela Džafić, Sanja Oručević Žuljević

First published in London, United Kingdom, 2022 by IntechOpen
IntechOpen is the global imprint of INTECHOPEN LIMITED, registered in England and Wales, registration number: 11086078, 5 Princes Gate Court, London, SW7 2QJ, United Kingdom

British Library Cataloguing-in-Publication Data
A catalogue record for this book is available from the British Library

Additional hard and PDF copies can be obtained from orders@intechopen.com

Pseudocereals
Edited by Viduranga Y. Waisundara
p. cm.
Print ISBN 978-1-80355-180-7
Online ISBN 978-1-80355-181-4
eBook (PDF) ISBN 978-1-80355-182-1

For EU product safety concerns:
IN TECH d.o.o., Prolaz Marije Krucifikse Kozulić 3, 51000 Rijeka, Croatia,
info@intechopen.com or visit our website at intechopen.com.

Meet the editor

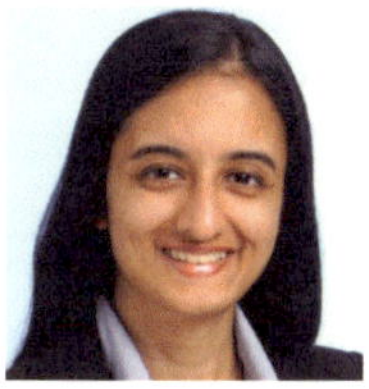

Dr. Viduranga Y. Waisundara obtained her Ph.D. in Food Science and Technology from the Department of Chemistry, National University of Singapore, in 2010. She was a lecturer at Temasek Polytechnic, Singapore from July 2009 to March 2013. She relocated to her motherland of Sri Lanka and spearheaded the Functional Food Product Development Project at the National Institute of Fundamental Studies from April 2013 to October 2016. She was a senior lecturer on a temporary basis at the Department of Food Technology, Faculty of Technology, Rajarata University of Sri Lanka. She is currently Deputy Principal of the Australian College of Business and Technology – Kandy Campus, Sri Lanka. She is also the Global Harmonization Initiative (GHI)

Contents

Preface

There are many kinds of cereal and grains that were consumed by our ancestors that could potentially provide solutions to issues of food and nutrition insecurity around the world. Within this context, a pseudocereal can be defined as one of any non-grasses that are used in much the same way as cereals (true cereals are grasses). Like any other cereal, the seed of a pseudocereal can be ground into flour and otherwise used as cereals. In ancient times, these pseudocereals served as staples for many civilizations because they were able to withstand harsh weather conditions, thus having the potential to curb any gaps and voids in the food supply chain throughout the year.

This book provides an overview of pseudocereals, including information on their nutritional value and processing techniques.

I would like to extend my appreciation to the contributing authors for their many wonderful chapters. Also, my heartfelt appreciation goes to IntechOpen with whom I have worked on many book projects. Finally, I wish to thank Publishing Process Manager Ms. Jasna Bozic who provided valuable support throughout the preparation and publication of this book.

With so many crisis situations around the world, it is my sincere hope that those who are interested and involved in doing research and investigations on pseudocereals will find this book to be a valuable resource. I also hope that the scientific community will come to view pseudocereals as a means of combating the global food crisis.

Dr. Viduranga Y. Waisundara
Deputy Principal,
Australian College of Business and Technology – Kandy Campus,
Kandy, Sri Lanka

Chapter 1

Introductory Chapter: Nutritive Value of Pseudocereals

Asel C. Weerasekera, Kanchana Samarasinghe and Viduranga Y. Waisundara

1. Introduction

Pseudocereals are becoming more popular in the gluten-free diet as a healthy substitute for gluten-containing grains in the modern world. The United States of America was the first country to recognize the health benefits of whole grains and embrace whole grains for the prevention of cancer and numerous cardiac diseases [1]. Grains are considered as an essential part of the human diet since the ancient time as it provides around 50% of an individual's energy and protein requirements (**Figure 1**).

2. Quinoa

This plant adjusts readily to many climate zones, agroecological soil types, and is a water-efficient crop that thrives in low-moisture environments [2]. Quinoa has a higher protein content than rice, making it more nutritious and it is also considered high in sugars such as R ribose, D galactose, and maltose [1]. It also contains an exceptional ratio of amino acids that are essential. It is abundant in phytosterols, saponins, and phytoecdysteroids, all of which are helpful for the overall quality of human health [3]. Moreover, albumin and globulin make up majority of the stored proteins in quinoa. Quinoa is considered to have high levels of non-protein tryptophan, which can be rapidly absorbed and helps to boost the usefulness of that kind of amino acid in the brain, influencing serotonin neurotransmitter production. Quinoa is low in saturated fats, rich in fiber, cholesterol-free, low in sodium, lowers the probability of

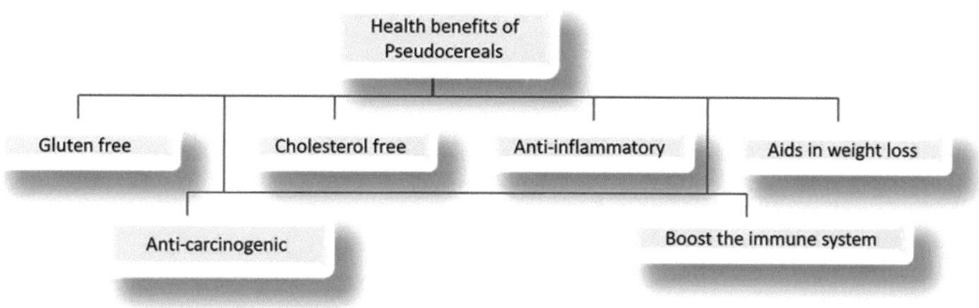

Figure 1.
Health benefits of Pseudocereals.

IntechOpen

forming kidney stones and gallbladder stones, helps digestion, and is high in antioxidants. Quinoa is rich in vitamin E, vitamin C and vitamin B [4]. Quinoa contains several phytochemicals that are produced through metabolism [5]. Cooked quinoa leaves are highly nutritious and easy to digest, and these leaves are consumed in most parts of the world to obtain various health benefits [6].

3. Amaranth

Amaranth plant is generally a fast-growing dicotyledonous plant that adapts to a wide range of soil types and climatic conditions. Amaranth is classed as a nutritious Pseudocereal due to its high protein content [7]. It is thought to have originated from the United States of America in the ancient time. However, Amaranth is now produced in most parts of the world since it is regarded as a superior pseudocereal with numerous health benefits. Amaranth aids in maintaining healthy cholesterol levels, Amaranth is also low in sodium, low in fats, aids in weight loss, anticarcinogenic and gluten free. Plant proteins found in amaranth include globulin, albumin, prolamins, and glutelin. Quinoa and Amaranth both pseudocereals are rich in folic acids. According to [6] when comparing normal cereals with pseudocereals, normal cereals contain low folic acids than pseudocereals. Amaranth is typically consumed as a popped cereal in the world and amaranth is also used as a flour to make types of pasta, bread and other food products [7]. Amaranth contains a lot of calcium and iron making it rich in nutritional values [8]. Amaranth is consumed by a number of individuals including athletes, individuals suffering from type 2 diabetes, people suffering from coeliac diseases and malnourished pupils (**Figure 2**).

4. Buckwheat

Buckwheat noodles and pasta are commonly consumed by people across the world at present. People consume buckwheat seeds primarily. In addition, buckwheat leaves are also consumed because of the health advantages [2]. Buckwheat, which is high in resistant starch, can help to reduce colon cancer. Buckwheat is rich in protein, several vitamins and unsaturated fats. Albumin and globulin are abundant in buckwheat [6] (**Figure 3**).

Due to the fiber content found in buckwheat, it has the capacity to lower blood lipid levels and to protect against chronic illnesses [9]. Some of the flavonoid compounds found in buckwheat include rutin, hyperin, procyanidin B-2, orientin, vitexin, quercetin, isovitexin, and kaempferol 1–2-0-rutinoside [9].

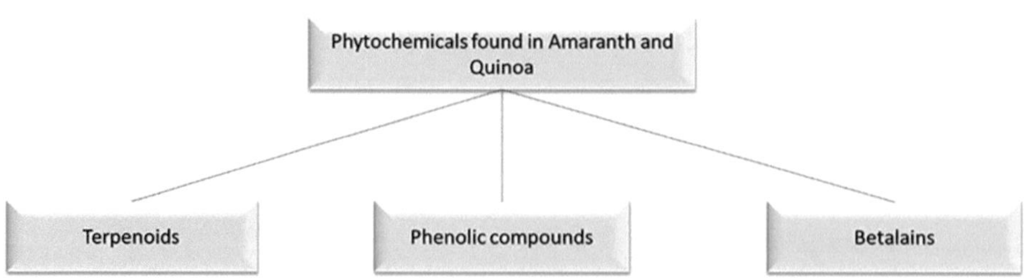

Figure 2.
Some of the phytochemicals that are common to Amaranth and Quinoa.

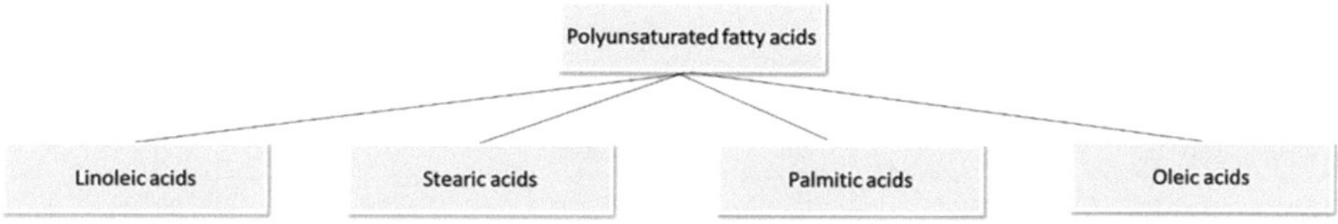

Figure 3.
Some of the polyunsaturated fatty acids present in buckwheat.

5. Millets

Millets are small-seeded crops of many species that are commonly produced in India to meet the production of food needed for a growing population. Millets are rich in nutrients and provide a number of health advantages. Different species of millets include Finger millet, Pearl millet, Foxtail millet, Little millet, Kodo millet and Barnyard millet. Millet is considered as a versatile grain that can be consumed in a variety of ways, including porridge, bread, beverages, and malt [10]. Millets contain significant amount of tryptophan, methionine, aromatic amino acids and cystine. Origin of millet is considered to be in Asia and in Northern Africa. Millets have the ability to reduce the risk of myocardial infarction, reduce diabetes, decrease high blood pressure, aids in maintaining healthy sleep routines, optimize kidneys, promote bone health and improve alkalinity. Millets are also gluten free and helps in relieving menstrual cramps in females.

5.1 Finger millet

Among the species of millet, Finger millet has a number of names that are used in different parts of the world (**Table 1**). The common finger millet is also called as *Eleusine coracana* in botanical terms [11].

5.2 Pearl millet

Around 500 million people across the world rely on pearl millet consumption and production for a living [10]. Pearl millet is a simple plant to grow compared to other grains. Pearl millet is known in the botanical name as *Pennisetum typhoides* and it also known in different names in different countries (**Table 2**).

Country	Name/s
India	Ragi
Saudi Arabia	Tailabon
Uganda	Bulo
Sri Lanka	Kurakkan
France	Koracan, *Eleusine coracana*
Germany	Fingerhirse

Table 1.
Alternative names used for finger millet by different countries across the world.

Country	Name/s
India	Bajra, Cumbu
Saudi Arabia	Dukhon
Nigeria	Gero
Sri Lanka	Muthu Meneri
France	mil du Soudan

Table 2.
Alternative names used for pearl millet by different countries across the world.

Country	Name/s
Germany	Hirse
Sri Lanka	Thana Meneri
Russia	Mogara, Morapa
Nepal	Kaguno

Table 3.
Alternative names used for foxtail millet by different countries across the world.

5.3 Foxtail millet

The botanical term of Foxtail millet is *Setaria italica* [12]. In ancient China, Foxtail millet was widely cultivated [8]. Around the world Foxtail millet is also known in different names as follows (**Table 3**).

5.4 Little millet, barnyard millet and kodo millet

Group of minor millets include little millet, barnyard millet, and Kodo millet. The botanical term of little millet is known as *Panicum sumatrense* and it belongs to the Poaceae family [12]. As this plant adapts well to a variety of climatic zones, it is planted in different parts of the world including India, Malaysia and China [12]. Barnyard millet is known as *Echinochloa esculenta*. Two types of Barnyard millet are famous around the world. Japanese Barnyard millet also known as *Echinochloa crus-galli* is one of the types and the other type is the Indian Barnyard millet which is generally known as *Echinochloa colona* [12]. Among the species of millet, Kodo millet

Country	Name/s
India	Kodo, Arugu
Africa	African bastard millet
Pakistan	Mandal
Sri Lanka	Ammu Meneri
New Zealand	Dutch millet

Table 4.
Alternative names used for little millet by different countries across the world.

is another species that is known in different names across the world (**Table 4**). The botanical name of Kodo millet is known as *Paspalum scrobiculatum* [12].

At present, various available processing techniques that are available in the world Pseudocereals and cereals are used in the food industry to produce food rich in numerous health benefits and to promote the concept of nutritional food to the modern world. This way it also uplifts the forgotten or the lost culinary dishes that ancestors considered to consume in the ancient time to fulfill the daily food requirement needed in village families.

6. Molecules found in pseudocereals and associated health benefits

6.1 Phytosterols

Phytosterols have a capacity to lower both total and low-density lipoprotein (LDL) levels in food. In high bioavailable tests that contained phytosterols dissolved in oil or egg fat, or emulsified with aqueous solutions [13], consistent LDL lowering was observed. Esterification of phytosterols in long-chain fatty acids increased bioavailability significantly, prompting functional food combinations which contain margarine with phytosterol containing pseudocereals.

The inherent difficulty in extracting phytosterols from plant-based diets has made testing the effects of baseline deficiency in phytosterol levels on diets. As such, very few such clinical tests have been carried out effectively. A recent study indicated a 38% increase in cholesterol absorption when corn oil was purified of phytosterols. Re-addition of the natural phytosterols gave baseline absorption levels, suggesting the LDL content is lowered through phytosterol action.

6.2 Saponins

Saponins are natural surfactants. They exhibit anti-protozoal activity. For example, saponin plant extracts contain protective effects against leishmaniasis. They also exhibit anti-bacterial properties (mostly pronounced against Gram-positive bacteria) at high doses, carried out via way of membranolytic interactions. Saponins also exhibit both humoral and cell-mediated immune system stimulation. As such, they have been implemented as adjuvants in vaccines. While containing the ability to increase intestinal permeability. The emulsification and micelle formation from saponins are expected to increase fatty acid absorption. Ability to reduce blood cholesterol levels. The Masai people's low serum cholesterol levels are attributed to the high number of saponin-rich herbs added to their largely milk and meat-based diets [14].

6.3 Phytoecdysteroids

Phytoecdysteroids contain the potential to decrease the rate of skeletal muscle deterioration via its activity as a mild anabolic agent. The atrophy and muscular fibrosis associated with Sarcopenia can potentially be combated with the aforementioned mechanism of action. In addition to this, Phytoecdysteroids also exhibit potential ability to reduce hyperglycemia and type 2 diabetes. Additionally, plants which contain ecdysteroids were used in traditional ethnobotanical medicinal systems in treatment of osteoporosis. Phytoecdysteroids also contain the capacity to assist people with Seasonal affective disorders, alcohol, and narcotic withdrawals alongside other stress related conditions [15].

6.4 Albumin, chenopodin and lunasin

Albumin exhibits a significant role in fluid distribution throughout the body owing to its colloidal property. It provides a significant level of normal oncotic pressure in intravascular spaces. The abundance and composition of Albumin also support its capacity to act as a transport molecule, or a solute [16].

Chenopodin is the primary seed storage protein of quinoa, and exhibits ability to bind carbohydrates, hemagglutinates erythrocytes, and is resistant to gram-negative bacteria. Chenopodin also inhibits inflammation and pain in in vivo models. Lunasin is another peptide variant from quinoa which exhibits reactive oxygen species (ROS) scavenging activity and nitric oxide production inhibition [17].

6.5 Tryptophan

As mentioned above, tryptophan is an important precursor for serotonin and melatonin. Additionally, playing a role in protein synthesis and co-enzyme NAD and NADP storage. Tryptophan is bound to circulating albumin plasma in high levels and exhibits brain-centric functional importance. The essential nature of tryptophan and the high levels of its availability in quinoa make the pseudocereal grain a possible alternative to vegan and vegetarian diets [18].

6.6 Folate

Folates are compounds exhibiting activity like pteroylglutamic acid, acting as an anti-anemia and growth factor. They are essential in carbon transfer steps in several DNA and RNA nucleotides. Advanced folate deficiency levels can lead to macrocytic or megaloblastic anemic conditions, mucous membrane lesions and neural tube defects during pregnancy. There is possibility of it being associated with severe complications such as spontaneous abortions, hemorrhage, separation of placenta from the inner wall of the uterus before birth, and preeclampsia.

The second most prominent condition of folate deficiency is homocysteinemia. It has been linked in recent years to coronary artery disease and stroke. Additionally, being implicated in mental retardation, developmental defects, occlusive disorders, osteoporosis, and dislocated lenses in children, as well as ischemic heart disease. It is part of the trifecta of the B-complex vitamin group alongside riboflavin and vitamin B12. Moreover, high dietary intake of folate has been observed with a decreased risk of carcinoma in situ [19].

6.7 Quercetin and rutin

Rutin exhibits neuroprotective activity, cardioprotective activity, anti-obesity, and antioxidant activity. In addition, rutin can be a potential adjuvant in radioiodine therapy, and shows ability to prevent or decrease the rate of age induced DNA fragmentation caused by apoptosis by inhibiting DNase I. Furthermore, it demonstrates ability to reduce lipid peroxidation in human sperm, contributing to combating male infertility [20]. Rutin has also been associated with lowering risks of arteriosclerosis, capillary fragility, and increased blood pressure. Other beneficial factors include restorative effects on renal diseases, possibly due to the combination of rutin, quercetin, hyperoside and phenolic oligomers found in buckwheat extracts used in studies. It also shows protective effects against gastric lesions and potential to be effective as a DNA protective component in the human diet [21, 22].

6.8 Hyperin

Hyperin exhibits antioxidant, anticancer, antiviral, anti-inflammatory, anti-bacterial, antiparasitic activity, cardio protective attributes, hepatoprotective attributes, anti-histamic, antifungal, apoptosis-inducing and anti-tumor abilities. Hyperin is also important in combating degenerative disease prevention associated with ROS [23].

6.9 Orientin

Orientin exhibits antioxidant activity, antiviral and antibacterial activity, anti-inflammatory activity, vasodilatory and cardioprotective effects, radioprotective effects, neuroprotection, and antidepressant activity, antiadipogenesis (undifferentiated precursor cells differentiating into fat cells) and, antinociceptive activity [24].

6.10 Vitexin and isovitexin

Vitexin and Isovitexin exhibit anticancer ability, anti-hypertensive ability, antidiabetic activity, anti-neoplastic effects, anti-inflammatory effects, protection against hypoxia and ischemia injury, protection against Alzheimer's disease, protective effects on learning, anti-depressive qualities, increasing levels of cerebral blood flow, anti-nociceptive activity, anti-convulsant effects, antiepileptic effects, anti-thyroid effects, anxiolytic properties, protection against endocrine and metabolic diseases, alongside anti-microbial and anti-viral effects [25].

6.11 Kaempferol

Kaempferol is a polyphenol antioxidant which has beneficial effects such as reducing risk of cancer, inducing cancer cell apoptosis, angiogenesis, anti-inflammation, anti-metastatic properties, and preservation of normal cell viability. Kaempferols have also been the target of recent nanoparticle coating to increase bioavailability due to the low natural occurrence of the substance in vivo. This is due to its poor dissolution in many solvents. However, the clinical properties encourage nanoparticle coating and investigation of the nano-chemopreventive aspect of kaempferol in patients, and further randomized, double blind, clinical testing [26].

7. Conclusion

As an Introductory chapter to this book, it is hoped that the readers will recognize the importance of the cereals highlighted herein and see them as means of imparting nutritive properties and health benefits. In times of trouble, it is possible that nutritionists and food technologists alike would have to look into the past and sought assistance from native grains and cereals which have enabled our ancestors to receive their nourishment. It is only through history that we can learn and un-learn our practices to look forth into a brighter future.

Author details

Asel C. Weerasekera[1], Kanchana Samarasinghe[2] and Viduranga Y. Waisundara[2*]

1 Western Sydney University, Sydney, Australia

2 Australian College of Business and Technology – Kandy Campus, Kandy, Sri Lanka

*Address all correspondence to: viduranga@gmail.com

References

[1] Greene SL, Williams KA, Khoury CK, Kantar MB, Marek LF. North American Crop Wild Relatives. Vol. Vol. 2. Cham, Switzerland: Springer; 2018

[2] Haros CM, Schoenlechner R, editors. Pseudocereals: Chemistry and Technology. UK: John Wiley & Sons; 2017

[3] Navruz-Varli S, Sanlier N. Nutritional and health benefits of quinoa (*Chenopodium quinoa* Willd.). Journal of Cereal Science. 2016;**69**:371-376

[4] Tang Y, Tsao R. Phytochemicals in quinoa and amaranth grains and their antioxidant, anti-inflammatory, and potential health beneficial effects: A review. Molecular Nutrition & Food Research. 2017;**61**(7):1600767

[5] Martínez JH, Velázquez F, Burrieza HP, Martínez KD, Rubio AP, dos Santos FC, et al. Betanin loaded nanocarriers based on quinoa seed 11S globulin. Impact on the protein structure and antioxidant activity. Food Hydrocolloids. 2019;**87**:880-890

[6] Thakur P, Kumar K, Dhaliwal HS. Nutritional facts, bio-active components and processing aspects of pseudocereals: A comprehensive review. Food Bioscience. 2021;**1**:101170

[7] Tovar-Pérez EG, Lugo-Radillo A, Aguilera-Aguirre S. Amaranth grain as a potential source of biologically active peptides: A review of their identification, production, bioactivity, and characterization. Food Reviews International. 2019;**35**(3):221-245

[8] Singh M, Sood S, editors. Millets and Pseudo Cereals: Genetic Resources and Breeding Advancements. Sawston, UK: Woodhead Publishing; 2020. DOI: 10.1016/C2019-0-00695-4

[9] Liangli LY, Tsao R, Shahidi F, editors. Cereals and Pulses: Nutraceutical Properties and Health Benefits. New York, USA: John Wiley & Sons; 2012

[10] National Research Council. Lost Crops of Africa: Volume I: Grains. Washington, DC: The National Academies Press. 1996. DOI: 10.17226/2305.

[11] Preedy VR, Watson RR, editors. Nuts and Seeds in Health and Disease Prevention. Cambridge, Massachusetts, USA: Academic Press; 2020. DOI: 10.1016/C2018-0-03983-3

[12] Singh M, Upadhyaya HD. Genetic and genomic resources for grain cereals improvement. Cambridge, Massachusetts, USA: Academic Press; 2015

[13] Ostlund RE Jr. Phytosterols in human nutrition. Annual Review of Nutrition. 2002;**22**(1):533-549

[14] Cheeke PR. Actual and potential applications of *Yucca schidigera* and *Quillaja saponaria saponins* in human and animal nutrition. In: Oleszek W, Marston A, editors. Saponins in Food, Feedstuffs and Medicinal Plants. Dordrecht: Springer; 2000. pp. 241-254

[15] Dinan L, Mamadalieva NZ, Lafont R. Dietary phytoecdysteroids. Handbook of Dietary Phytochemicals. Singapore: Springer; 2019:1-54. DOI: 10.1007/978-981-13-1745-3_35-1

[16] Doweiko JP, Nompleggi DJ. Reviews: Role of albumin in human physiology and pathophysiology. Journal of Parenteral and Enteral Nutrition. 1991 Mar;**15**(2):207-211

[17] Pompeu DG, Cordeiro HG, Tonelli FC, Godin AM, Melo IS,

Matsui TC, et al. Chenopodin as an anti-inflammatory compound. Natural Product Research. 2021;**13**:1-4

[18] Comai S, Bertazzo A, Bailoni L, Zancato M, Costa CV, Allegri G. The content of proteic and nonproteic (free and protein-bound) tryptophan in quinoa and cereal flours. Food Chemistry. 2007;**100**(4):1350-1355

[19] Krishnaswamy K, Nair KM. Importance of folate in human nutrition. British Journal of Nutrition. 2001; **85**(S2):S115-S124

[20] Kolarevic A, Pavlovic A, Djordjevic A, Lazarevic J, Savic S, Kocic G, et al. Rutin as deoxyribonuclease I inhibitor. Chemistry & Biodiversity. 2019;**16**(5):e1900069

[21] Kreft I, Fabjan N, Germ M. Rutin in buckwheat-protection of plants and its importance for the production of functional food. Fagopyrum. 2003;**20**(7):7-11

[22] Nabavi SF, Russo GL, Daglia M, Nabavi SM. Role of quercetin as an alternative for obesity treatment: you are what you eat! Food Chemistry. 2015;**179**:305-310

[23] Patel K, Kumar V, Rahman M, Verma A, Patel DK. New insights into the medicinal importance, physiological functions and bioanalytical aspects of an important bioactive compound of foods 'Hyperin': Health benefits of the past, the present, the future. Beni-Suef University Journal of Basic and Applied Sciences. 2018;7(1):31-42

[24] Peng Y, Gan R, Li H, Yang M, McClements DJ, Gao R, et al. Absorption, metabolism, and bioactivity of vitexin: Recent advances in understanding the efficacy of an important nutraceutical. Critical Reviews in Food Science and Nutrition. 2021;**61**(6):1049-1064

[25] He M, Min JW, Kong WL, He XH, Li JX, Peng BW. A review on the pharmacological effects of vitexin and isovitexin. Fitoterapia. 2016;**115**:74-85

[26] Chen AY, Chen YC. A review of the dietary flavonoid, kaempferol on human health and cancer chemoprevention. Food Chemistry. 2013;**138**(4):2099-2107

Chapter 2

Use of Common Buckwheat in the Production of Baked and Pasta Products

Tatiana Bojňanská, Alena Vollmannová, Judita Lidiková and Janette Musilová

Abstract

This chapter introduces buckwheat as a possible raw material for the production of designed foods. It includes the description of common buckwheat as a source of basic nutrients for food production and gives specificities of buckwheat as a source of biologically active substances. Processed buckwheat seeds are important from the point of view of rational nutrition as a source of energy, carbohydrates, fibre, proteins, lipids, vitamins, and minerals. Buckwheat has also other nutritional advantages, especially the interesting content of polyphenolic compounds: phenolic acids, flavonoids, especially rutin, which are characterised by high antioxidant activity. This chapter describes how buckwheat can be processed into food products and discusses the results of the application of buckwheat to bread and pasta. Moreover, it includes the results of the clinical study. Based on the identified technological and sensory properties of bread products obtained during the baking experiment, the chapter summarises recommendations on the suitable added amount of buckwheat to get satisfactory results. Concerning pasta from buckwheat, it had very good technological, nutritional, and sensory qualities. The chapter concludes that, on the basis of findings, buckwheat is a raw material suitable for the production of designed foods.

Keywords: common buckwheat, polyphenolic compounds, technological properties, dough rheology, rheofermentometer, bread quality, pasta properties

1. Introduction

The sustainable development of agriculture is based, among other things, on the efficient use of gene funds. The use of species or varieties with high resistance, high yield stability, the ability to use nutrients efficiently and high nutritional quality is a guarantee of biodiversity conservation extending and intensifying the use of species and varietal diversity to less grown crops, whether traditional or forgotten, can bring new types of products with the higher nutritional quality or added value. This is also one of the ways how to innovate existing foods. Presently, there is a growing interest in such crops.

Without any doubt, buckwheat is one of these interesting raw materials. It is included among pseudocereals, which botanically do not belong to cereals, but their use is similar. It comes from Southeast Asia, the first written records of the plant are in Chinese documents of the fifth and sixth century AD. It came to Europe from Russia in the Middle Ages, and in the territory of today's Slovakia, it began to be grown in the thirteenth–fourteenth century [1]. For many centuries it was a vital food source for the inhabitants of mountainous regions where the climate is cold and the soil is poor [2]. It belongs to the family Polygonaceae, to the genus *Fagopyrum*. *Fagopyrum esculentum* (Moench) and *Fagopyrum tataricum* (L.) Gaertn can be grown for grain yield (*Fagopyri semen*), with the most important species being *Fagopyrum esculentum*. It is an annual plant 0.5–2 m high, branched at the top. The flowers are white, white-pink, and sometimes red, they bloom gradually from bottom to top and are foreign-pollinated, mainly by bees. The fruit of buckwheat is a triangular smooth achene (seeds of a curious shape, triangular in cross-section with pointed ends) with a brown to violet-red colour. The potential yield is 1.5–2.5 t/ha [3, 4]. It can also be used as fodder or honey plant. Buckwheat stems and leaves (*Fagopyri herba*), which were previously used only as animal feed, are currently also used for human consumption. Buckwheat was once a widely grown crop in Central Europe, but was gradually replaced by more intensive species. So it can be described as a "forgotten" crop. Buckwheat's renaissance is motivated mainly by health reasons.

In terms of nutrition, buckwheat seeds have a very favourable composition. Properly processed and modified buckwheat seeds are important from the point of view of rational nutrition as a source of energy, carbohydrates, fibre, vitamins, lipids, and minerals. Especially proteins of buckwheat seeds are valuable thanks to their composition which makes buckwheat suitable for food production for celiacs.

Buckwheat also has other nutritional advantages, especially the interesting content of polyphenolic compounds: phenolic acids, flavonoids, especially rutin, which are characterised by high antioxidant activity. Taking into consideration all characteristics, buckwheat is a raw material suitable for the production of designed foods [5, 6].

2. Common buckwheat as a source of basic nutrients for food production

This section gives an overview of buckwheat's seeds composition referring to the content of important nutrients, namely, proteins, fibre, amino acids, starch, fats as well as minerals. For food production, the dehulled seeds, called the groats, are the preferred used part of buckwheat. They are rich in proteins, their content in buckwheat groats is around 12% and more, and their biological value is relatively high [7]. Buckwheat protein contains a wide range of various amino acids, the most represented being glutamic acid, aspartic acid, and arginine. Of the essential amino acids, the content of lysine, leucine, valine, but also methionine and tryptophan is particularly important. Buckwheat can therefore serve as a natural plant source of these amino acids essential for the human body [8, 9]. Buckwheat proteins can be divided on the basis of their solubility into protein fractions, with the share of albumins and globulins as the most valuable fractions being up to 50–65%, and a low proportion of prolamin proteins (3–6%), which makes buckwheat a suitable raw material also for celiacs [9, 10]. In buckwheat, 13S globulin and 8S globulin have been identified, where 13S globulin contributes to 33% of total seeds proteins and is a major storage protein [11]. Most of the protein in buckwheat is localised in protein bodies.

The main proportion of carbohydrates found in buckwheat seeds consists mainly of starch, the content of which varies in a relatively wide range from 58 to 70%. This may be due to genetically fixed characteristics of the variety, agro-ecological cultivation conditions or climatic conditions. Buckwheat starch granule sizes are 2.9–9.3 μm with an average size of 5.8 μm and have a round or polygonical shape [9].

In addition to starch as an energy source, there is also the potential for resistant starch in buckwheat [12]. Resistant starch is a portion of starch and starch degraded products that escape enzymatic hydrolysis in the small intestine. There are indications that metabolites formed during the fermentation of resistant starch in the large intestine, contribute to the maintenance of colon health and have beneficial effects on glucose metabolism as well. For most healthy adults, consuming foods with a higher amount of resistant starch is, therefore, advantageous. Undigested starch may result in positive nutritional effects that are similar to effects observed with fibre [12]. Besides, foods with higher levels of resistant starch usually have a low GI (Glycaemic Index).

Moreover, buckwheat is rich in dietary fibre that has a positive physiological effect on the gastrointestinal tract and significantly influences the metabolism of other nutrients. Dietary fibre can be divided into insoluble fibre and soluble fibre. In buckwheat seeds, hemicellulose is the predominant fraction, while in buckwheat hulls lignin and cellulose are dominant [13]. In buckwheat seeds dietary fibre constitutes from 5 to 11%, the soluble fraction content is around 3–7%, while the amount of the insoluble fraction is approx. 2–4% [8]. The physiological effect of dietary fibre depends first of all on its origin, the proportions of individual fractions, the degree of comminution of raw materials and the applied thermal processes. The insoluble fraction of dietary fibre (generally includes lignin and cellulose) that activates the intestinal peristalsis is capable of binding bile acids and water. Soluble fibre (includes pectin and gums) reduces the blood cholesterol level, the risk of incidence of ischemic heart disease and postprandial glycaemia. The functional properties of dietary fibre, such as water holding capacity, cation binding, and sorption of bile acids, play a significant role in the prevention of diet-dependent diseases, e.g. obesity, atherosclerosis, and colon cancer [14]. However, dietary fibre can also have a negative role as it may bind proteins and minerals, inhibit digestive enzymes, and thereby lower digestibility or absorption.

With regards to the content of fats, achenes of buckwheat contain 2–3% of fats that are concentrated in the embryo. In buckwheat flour, the embryo is generally included (mostly in bran fraction), so the content of fats in groats and flour is 3–4% [15], and the risk of deterioration by lipids is therefore particularly important. Oleic acid is the dominant unsaturated fatty acid (≈33%) in the seed oil, followed by linoleic acid (≈32%), which belongs to the essential fatty acids and has many physiological functions. The main saturated fatty acid is palmitic acid (≈13%). Stearic acid (≈1.6%) and others are also present in smaller amounts [16].

As for the content of important minerals in buckwheat, it is also substantial, especially since the levels of Mg, Zn, K, P, Fe, Cu, and Mn are high when compared to cereals. For example, Mg, Zn, K, P, and Co are mainly stored as phytate in the protein bodies. Minerals such as Fe, Zn, Mn, Cu, Mo, Ni, and Al are primarily located in both the hull and seed coat [17]. The largest difference between the content of a particular mineral element in groats compared to seeds, is found with Ca (more than a fourfold decrease), Fe (more than a threefold decrease), and Mn (one and a half fold decrease) [18].

Buckwheat, therefore, provides all the important sources of basic nutrients for food production, and in addition, its great advantage is the presence of biologically active substances, which generally affect the physiological processes in the body of consumers in the desired.

3. Common buckwheat as a source of biologically active substances

As illustrated above, buckwheat has a favourable composition of the protein complex, fibre content, and minerals. In addition, it contains also vitamins as well as phytochemicals with a prophylactic value and biological activity as presented in this section. Here, we also describe which compounds are found in different parts of a buckwheat plant.

Vitamins are a group of organic compounds that are essential in very small amounts for the normal functioning of the human body. Group B vitamins are very important components of the vitamin complex contained in buckwheat: B1 (thiamine), B2 (riboflavin), B3 (niacin), B5 (pantothenic acid), B6 (pyridoxine). Other vitamins present are vitamin C in buckwheat sprouts, and vitamin E (tocopherols). In buckwheat seeds, thiamine is strongly adhered to thiamine-binding proteins [6, 9]. An important component of the vitamin complex in buckwheat is choline, an essential nutrient, and choline esters that are potential functional food ingredients. Choline is used by the body for the biosynthesis of phospholipids and acetylcholine, which is used in the transmission of nerve impulses. It is also used therapeutically for liver damage. The daily requirement is about 600 mg. In 1 kg of common buckwheat seeds on a dry matter basis (dry weight/d.w.), the content is about 440 mg [19].

A larger proportion of phenolic compounds in buckwheat are flavonoids. Flavonoids are classified into numerous subgroups, namely, flavonols, flavones, flavanones, flavanols, anthocyanins, fagopyrins, proanthocyanidins, isoflavones, and flavonolignans. The major flavonoids in buckwheat are rutin, quercetin, orientin, homoorientin, vitexin, kaempferol, and isovitexin. Different types of flavonoids have been detected in the root, leaves, flower, seed, sprouted seed, seed coat, seed husk, and processed food of buckwheat [20]. Flavonoid compounds present in buckwheat are significantly important to improve human health and to prevent and heal different diseases [6].

Almost all parts of buckwheat are the source of many health beneficial components, however, the differences in the content of polyphenolic substances found in different anatomic parts (stems, leaves, flowers, and seeds) are significant. The concentration of flavonoids and main phenolic acids was monitored in the flowers, seeds, and leaves [21–24]. The highest concentration of chlorogenic acid and *trans*-sinapic acid was found in the flowers. For other studied phenolics, the highest concentration was established in the leaves, followed by the flowers and then the seeds [24].

The flavonoids content and composition in buckwheat seeds is affected by cultivar, location, growing phase, and growing conditions. When evaluating the dynamics of the total polyphenols formation, the maximum increase in the polyphenolic contents was observed during the full ripeness growing phase. The highest polyphenol content was found in the leaves, followed by the seeds and stems (there were no more flowers in this growing phase) [25]. Different polyphenol contents were also found in common buckwheat cultivars [26] and the determining role of the cultivar on the relative content of chlorogenic acid, *trans*-caffeic acid, *trans*-sinapic acid, vitexin, and kaempferol in buckwheat plants was confirmed. The content of the dominant flavonoid rutin in the seeds of buckwheat cultivars (8) varied in the range from 2.791 mg/g d.w. (cv. Pulawska, Poland) to 13.326 mg/g d.w. (cv. Ballada, Russia) [24].

The most important flavonoid in buckwheat is rutin, which has remarkable effects on the human organism. It reduces high blood pressure, the risk of arteriosclerosis, and has also antioxidant activity [5, 27]. Rutin is also used medicinally in many countries to reduce capillary fragility associated with some haemorrhagic diseases in humans. In 1 kg of buckwheat seed on a dry matter basis, there is approximately 60–80 g of rutin [24], which is an important amount, but this might decrease due to the culinary preparation (cooking). It is also necessary to take into account the distribution of rutin and possibly other flavonoids in buckwheat seeds according to the milling fractions during the milling process. In common buckwheat, rutin is mainly located in the hull, and its concentration is low in groats or flours (**Figures 1** and **2**) [21–26, 28].

All polyphenols are reducing agents, and as such, they may scavenge free radicals and protect cell constituents against oxidative damage. Especially flavonoids belong to the plant components with an antioxidant activity, which is a fundamental property important for life. The differences in the chemical structures of different flavonoids affect their antioxidant activities. Buckwheat appears to be a suitable component of food products with regard to its nutritional aspect and its antioxidant activity [29]. A significant relationship between the total phenolic as well as rutin content in common buckwheat and antioxidant activity was found [30]. The antioxidant activity differences were also found between buckwheat cultivars as well as among the different parts of the plant [31].

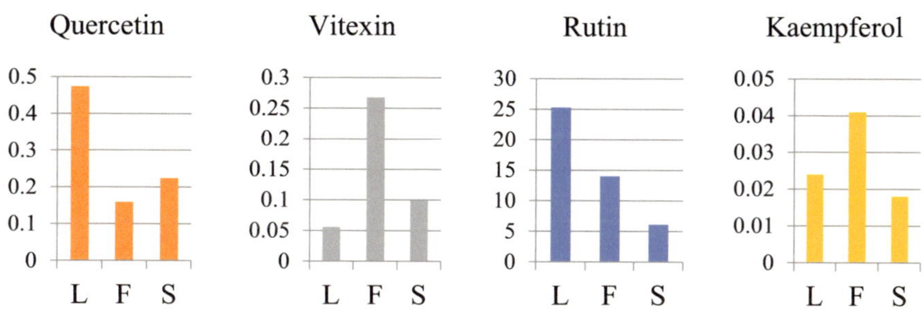

Figure 1.
Graphical overview of differences in flavonoids content in different parts of common buckwheat: L (leaves), F (flowers), S (seeds).

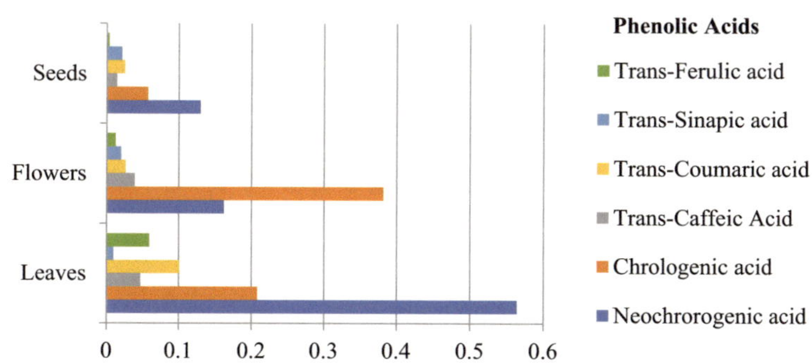

Figure 2.
Graphical overview of differences in phenolic acids content in different parts of common buckwheat: L (leaves), F (flowers), S (seeds).

The use of buckwheat in food production, and not just seeds but also other parts of the plant, can improve the nutritional value of foods thanks to adding an antioxidant activity from natural sources. However, the safety and toxicity profiles of the roots, leaves, and hulls of buckwheat have not been completely analysed until now. There may be some risks associated with eating buckwheat. Buckwheat parts, leaves, in particular, contain fagopyrins, phototoxic phenolic substances belonging to the group anthraquinones. When fagopyrins accumulate under the skin, it causes fagopyrism, which manifests itself when the skin is exposed to sunlight. Fagopyrism has been described in the past in livestock, which feeds on buckwheat leaves. The seeds contain very few fagopyrins but the whole plant, either dried or green, can cause serious problems potentially also for people, because of the consumption of buckwheat leaves, e.g. through the juice from the leaves [9, 32, 33].

The possibility of buckwheat allergy should be also mentioned. This is a clinical condition known for a long time and is frequent in Asia, where this crop is commonly eaten. An allergy to buckwheat is typically IgE mediated, several buckwheat proteins are described as being able to bind IgE in allergic patients. Proteins with a molecular weight of 9, 16, 19, and 24 kDa are considered major allergens [34]. In Europe, buckwheat allergy was not documented until a few years ago, when the consumption of buckwheat increased. Buckwheat allergy merits awareness in Europe since exposures are likely to increase via the use of buckwheat as it is becoming popular in the food sector. Failure to recognise buckwheat allergy could expose individuals to a considerable risk. A particular aspect of allergic reactions to buckwheat reported in Europe is that they are often severe and systemic, such as anaphylaxis, and often triggered by buckwheat not declared in dishes that are not supposed to contain it [35].

Despite these risks, and based on a comprehensive consideration of nutritional benefits, buckwheat appears to be an excellent raw material for food processing, which is described in the next section.

4. Food processing of buckwheat

For food production, the most usable part of buckwheat is achene, which is covered on the surface with a hard dark hull. Before processing the achenes, they must be separated without damaging the endosperm. Currently, two basic technological processes are used in the world for dehulling buckwheat, namely, mechanical dehulling and thermal dehulling. It must be taken into consideration that dehulling the seeds by using different temperature regimens results in drastic reductions of the total flavonoid concentration in the seeds (by 75% of the control) [36], thus, reducing considerably the amount of positive substances. Dehulled seeds are further processed into buckwheat groats or buckwheat flour.

Buckwheat dishes have a long tradition and certain specifics must be taken into account in their cooking. In dry state, buckwheat is relatively hard, but it loses this property after receiving a sufficient amount of water or other liquid. In the process of swelling, buckwheat groats absorb water and double their volume. From a practical point of view, this means that each kilogramme of buckwheat groats receives 2.0–2.5 l of water. When boiling water is poured over buckwheat groats, they can be even served without cooking after cooling slowly in a sealed container. It should be noted that sufficient time for swelling buckwheat groats cannot be replaced by intense cooking. There might be certain disadvantages of buckwheat products, mainly the typical buckwheat aroma, which must be accepted. Also the possible odour after becoming musty, or acquired foreign odour could be perceptible as buckwheat is very prone to absorbing foreign odours [3]. A promising and unobtrusive way of how to apply buckwheat in food is its addition in the form of flour to other, often basic foods, for example, in bread, pastry, cakes, pancakes, biscuits, cookies, pasta, and noodles.

4.1 Application of common buckwheat to bread

As mentioned previously, the addition of buckwheat in basic food such as bread has proven to be a very convenient way of making bread more nutritionally attractive. This section describes the nutritional advantages of buckwheat additions in flours intended for the production of bread and pastries, but on the other hand, brings up the subject of the technological disadvantages.

Bread is food consumed on a daily basis and is generally very popular in the world. In Europe, bread is the main source of carbohydrates in the diet, but its consumption is on a declining trend. In Slovakia, for example, the consumption of bread and pastries (bread under 400 g) has fallen by almost 30 kg in the last 30 years, despite the nutritional recommendations, according to which the share of carbohydrates in the energy supply to the body should be 50–60%. In Slovakia, this recommended value according to age, gender, and work intensity ranges from ≈48% for infants, through ≈60% for adolescents (up to 18 years) and ≈58% for working adults [37].

Bread is an integral part of the diet, it contains essential nutrients, antioxidants, as well as vitamins. Even after thousands of years of consumption, it remains the most commonly consumed food in the world, also thanks to its readiness, portability, nutritional value, and taste [38]. Currently, however, carbohydrate foods are considered by the public to be a group of foods with a lower nutritional value. There are several reasons for this lower bread consumption, one of them being the increasing number of consumers who reject foods containing gluten, even if they do not have any health reasons (celiac disease, non-celiac sensitivity). One way to increase the proportion of biologically valuable ingredients in bread, and thus make it a more attractive food, is to partially replace the typical bread and rye bread raw materials with non-bakery raw materials, which are expected to meet consumer requirements for bioavailable and nutritionally necessary ingredients [39–41]. Buckwheat is undoubtedly such raw material.

However, due to the properties of non-bakery raw materials that do not meet the technological requirements, it is often a problem to prepare a product with the required volume, porosity, or sensory properties [42, 43]. From the technological and sensory point of view, the volume of bread or pastry is very important. The volume is ensured by the processes taking place during fermentation and the ability of the dough to retain the fermentation gases in the required volume. However, the addition of non-gluten raw materials weakens the dough due to the fact that they do not form the gluten nets, which affects the viscoelasticity of the dough, incorporation of air during kneading, and gas retention during fermentation. This process is resulting in bread with a weak structure and crumb texture [44, 45]. It is important to recognise that although from a nutritional point of view, the enriching addition should be as high as possible, from a technological and sensory point of view, an acceptable compromise must be found.

The bakery and non-bakery buckwheat products are prepared in many countries according to various often traditional recipes. The following part focuses on the possibilities of preparing enriched breads as a source of biologically active ingredients in nutrition. Buckwheat flour was mixed with wheat flour in different proportions (10, 20, 30, 40 and 50%). We present below the results of the suitability of using buckwheat flour in bakery products obtained by the available rheological instruments. We also carried out the baking test and gave possible suggestions on optimal amounts of buckwheat in bread. The raw materials used were not physically, chemically, or biologically treated to modify their technological properties, and were analysed for standard parameters of technological quality. The wheat flour used was good quality, strong flour with a high crude protein content (13% d.w.), with a good wet gluten content (25.6%), with an excellent swelling and adequate enzymatic activity (falling number 358 s). The buckwheat flour used had a slightly higher crude protein content (13.8%) and more than twice the ash content compared to wheat flour [46].

Measuring the rheological properties of dough intended for bread production is relatively complicated due to the exploitation of specific equipment. Rheology studies the relations between the tension a material is exposed to, the final dimension of material deformation and time. The rheological measurement is used to obtain a quantitative description of the material's mechanical properties and to get data with relation to its molecular structure and composition. It also enables to characterise and simulate the efficiency of the material during the production and the quality check [47, 48]. As part of rheological analyses (Farinograph-E, Extenzograph-E, Brabender) the changes in the physical properties of wheat flour and composite flours with the addition of buckwheat were monitored. The influence of buckwheat added to composite flours on the properties evaluated by a farinograph was significant [49, 50]. With an increasing portion of buckwheat, the dough consistency (in comparison to wheat flour) decreased, the dough became weaker and the resistance against the farinograph blades was lower (**Figure 3**).

Rheological properties of wheat dough affect mainly the gluten content and its qualitative properties. The high gluten swelling in wheat flour was beneficial since buckwheat does not contain gluten-forming proteins and reduces the gluten content in buckwheat-containing composite flours. This reduction in bread making causes technological problems, as gluten proteins play a key role in ensuring the baking quality of wheat and affect water binding, cohesion, viscosity, ductility, flexibility, stretch resistance, kneading tolerance as well as the ability to retain fermentation gases [51–53].

The rheological properties of dough changed when increasing the amount of buckwheat in the composite flour. The water absorption of dough decreased slightly when increasing the addition of buckwheat in the mixture, which is less desirable from an economic point of view, as the amount of flour needed to produce the same weight of dough increases. The farinograph curve confirmed the prolongation of the dough development time and increased energy input demands for kneading the dough with an optimal consistency by increasing the buckwheat addition.

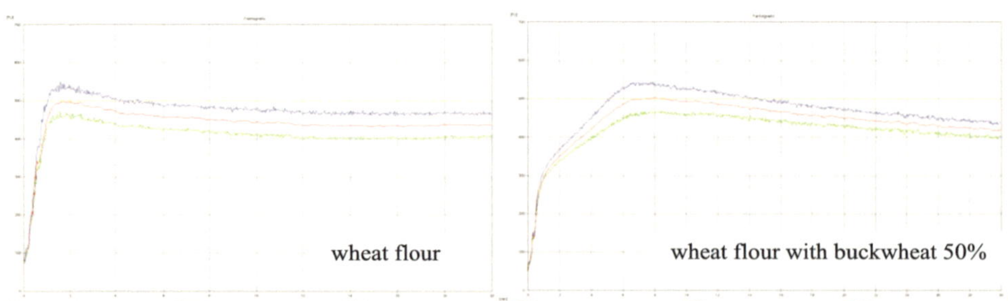

Figure 3.
Farinograph wheat flour and farinograph wheat flour with buckwheat 50%.

The development time of the dough with the addition of buckwheat 20% or more was considerably higher than in the control sample (9.0–9.5 min and 1.7 min, respectively) [43]. A longer dough development time is typical for bakery strong flours, but bakeries prefer flours with a shorter dough development because of the energy intensity of kneading. Subsequently, the behaviour of the dough with the addition of buckwheat was verified in different kneading modes. The Sigma blades of the farinograph worked with three different speeds (standard—63 revs./min, low—45 revs./min and high—120 revs./min). In composite flours with a higher proportion of buckwheat (20%<), the slow speed further prolonged the development time of the dough, but at high speed, the development time of the dough was already at the same level as in wheat flour. With the increasing addition of buckwheat, the extensographic energy (cm^2), extensographic resistance (BU Brabender unit), extensographic ductility (mm), as well as the ratio of resistance and ductility also decreased. With the increasing addition of buckwheat, the dough was less durable and unstable when kneading, which is a prerequisite for reducing the volume of bread [46, 54]. Therefore, when preparing dough with non-bakery raw materials, it is necessary to consider, verify and set the optimal kneading mode.

Determining the ability to form fermenting gases is crucial to produce bread with a good volume. To determine the rheofermentation properties a rheofermentometer Rheo F4 is used, by means of which the total volume of gas, the volume of gas lost, and the retention volume produced under the conditions of the method are determined. It is important to note that the produced CO_2 serves to expand the dough and achieve the final loaf volume. The unique properties of wheat flour to form a viscoelastic dough that can retain gas are due to the protein characteristics of wheat gluten when it is mixed with water [55]. Composite flours with buckwheat addition decrease the total amount of gluten, resulting in the formation of a weaker protein network. **Figure 4** clearly illustrates the CO_2 production during the fermentation of dough with an addition of buckwheat in a portion of 30%. In the dough with an addition of buckwheat, the gas production was more intensive. The total volume of gas in the composite flour dough was higher than in the wheat flour dough (1792 ml and 1408 ml, respectively), but the CO_2 losses in the composite flour dough were up to 2.6 times higher than in the wheat flour dough (580 ml and 219 ml, respectively), so finally the retention volume was at approximately the same level in both samples. This finding was positive and gave an assumption for an adequate volume of the final product—bread [47, 56, 57].

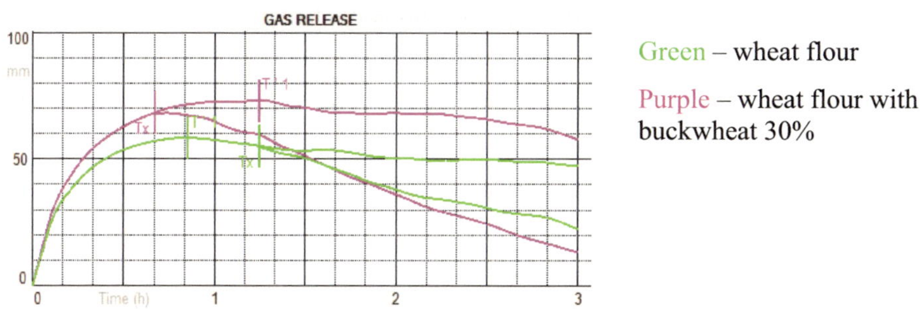

Figure 4.
Rheofermentometer curves of wheat flour and wheat + buckwheat composite flour.

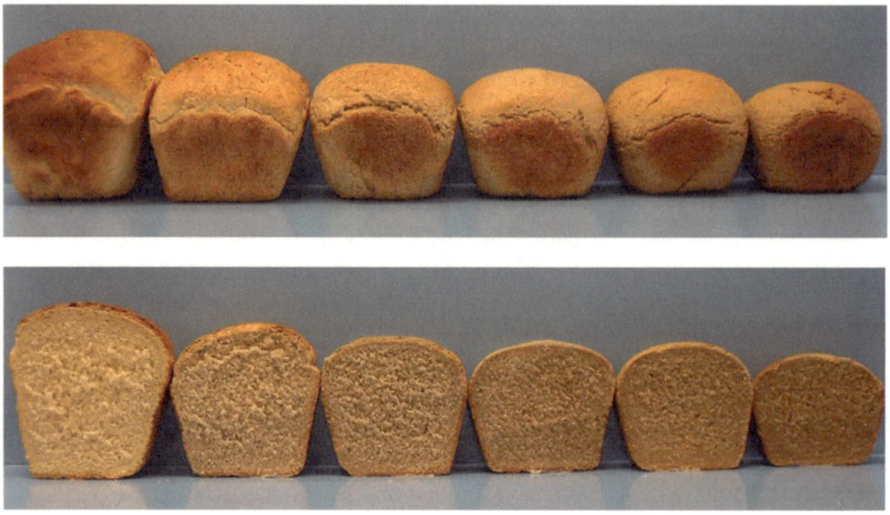

Figure 5.
Experimental breads with the addition of buckwheat (wheat bread > with 10% of buckwheat > with 20% of buckwheat > with 30% of buckwheat > with 40% of buckwheat > with 50% of buckwheat). Photo: author.

The baking test is the direct method for determining the quality of the applied raw materials and composite flours. During the baking process, the flour blends were subjected to mechanical work and heat treatment that promote changes in their physicochemical properties [58]. The final product has physical and sensory properties that make it a well-digestible and popular staple food. The experimental breads were prepared from composite flours with the addition of buckwheat in the amount of 10, 20, 30, 40 and 50%, water, salt, and yeast in the amount according to the recipe. They were baked according to the workplace methodologies in a steamed oven at a maximum temperature of 260°C [42, 46, 54]. Subsequently, they were subjected to evaluation by objective parameters and a sensory evaluation. Increasing the buckwheat amount in blends with wheat flour decreased the important parameters such as loaf volume, specific loaf volume, and volume efficiency (**Figure 5**). The same trend was observed for loaf arching, which is the ratio between height and width, and its higher value predicts a loaf with a more desirable, arched shape [59]. With the addition of buckwheat, the acidity of the crumb changed considerably. The acidity is an indicator of the content of acidic substances, or acids present in the starting material, but also formed during fermentation. Too low a value of titratable acids is not desirable, because such a pastry has a dull and unimpressive flavour. An increased crumb acidity can be considered desirable because of its distinctive flavour and taste during sensorial proofing.

The results of the sensory assessment of buckwheat-enriched breads show a gradual deterioration of most of the evaluated parameters depending on the amount of the addition. Although the addition of buckwheat did not have an important effect on the colour of the crust, it considerably intensified the colour of the crumb, the elasticity of which decreased when increasing the addition [50]. The colour of the bread crumb depends largely on the colour of the flour, the ash content, the presence of bran particles, the pore structure of the crumb and the way the dough is formed. The fineness of the crumb is directly related to the product volume, the pore structure, the additives used (emulsifiers, enzymes), the moisture content,

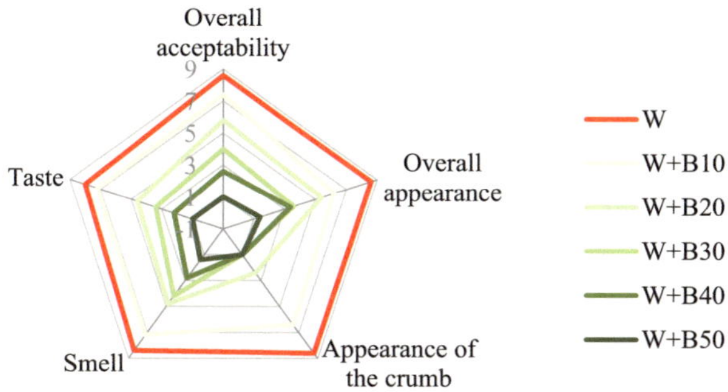

Figure 6.
Sensory profile of breads with the addition of buckwheat.

the baking conditions (time), and the storage conditions (temperature/time) [60, 61]. The appearance of the surface, the appearance of the crumb, the smell, the taste, and the overall acceptability expressed by the hedonic scale (0–9) are documented in **Figure 6**, from which the reduction in the point rating of these properties is evident [46]. Of all the loaves evaluated, the control loaf was the most acceptable (8.6) and the overall acceptability decreased with the amount of the addition: buckwheat addition of 10% (7.4) > buckwheat addition of 20% (5.8) > buckwheat addition of 30% (4.0) > buckwheat addition of 40% (2.6) > buckwheat addition of 50% (1.0).

W-common wheat flour, W + B10-common wheat flour + buckwheat wholegrain flour 10%, W + B20-common wheat flour + buckwheat wholegrain flour 20%, W + B30-common wheat flour + buckwheat wholegrain flour 30%, W + B40-common wheat flour + buckwheat wholegrain flour 40%, W + B50-common wheat flour + buckwheat wholegrain flour 50%.

From the consumer's point of view, the sensory acceptability of the product is especially important, so ultimately the organoleptic evaluation decides on its success on the market. Based on the results of measuring the physical properties of the dough and the baking experiment, the 10% buckwheat addition seems to be the most suitable. Such an addition did not significantly reduce the technological properties of the dough or pastry. Although higher buckwheat additions gave products with the expected higher nutritional value, they were technologically rated as worse, although still acceptable. We assume that technological shortcomings could be partially compensated by the use of suitable additives with improving properties. From the overall acceptability rating, it was concluded that bread with the addition of 10%, 20%, and 30% of buckwheat could be baked with satisfactory results. Such enriched bread is considered of a high nutritive value and acceptable from a sensory point of view, therefore, we can recommend these amounts of buckwheat additions as appropriate.

In general, the increasing addition of buckwheat worsens the technological and sensory parameters of bread compared to wheat bread, but on the other hand, there is an increase in nutritional value due to the content of valuable buckwheat components. The wheat bread contained 11.39% of protein, the acceptable addition of buckwheat at 30% increased the protein content to 13.63%, which is 17% more than in the control bread. The predominant protein fractions in buckwheat are albumin and globulin, rich in histidin, threonine, valine, phenylalanine, isoleucine and lysine [40, 62], which is undoubtedly a nutritional benefit. In such enriched bread the other important bioactive components (ash, fibre, vitamin B, rutin and antioxidant activity) increased as well [41, 63]. The rutin content in buckwheat wholegrain flour was 79.9 mg/kg (d.w.),

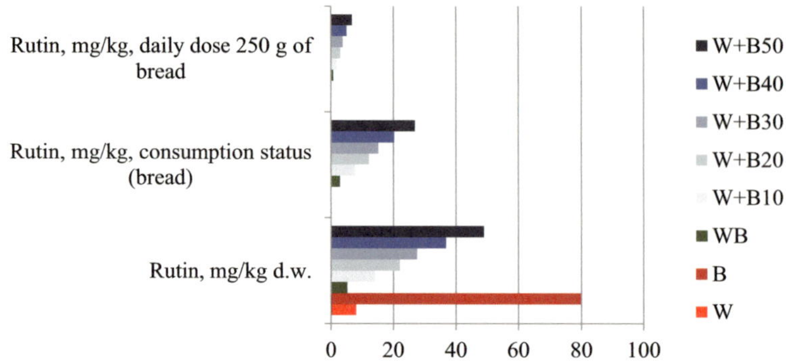

Figure 7.
Rutin content in bread (d.w., consumption status, daily dose). W-common wheat flour, B-buckwheat wholegrain flour, WB-wheat bread, W + B10-bread with 10% of buckwheat, W + B20-bread with 20% of buckwheat, W + B30-bread with 30% of buckwheat, W + B40-bread with 40% of buckwheat, W + B50-bread with 50% of buckwheat.

in wheat flour it was 8.1 mg/kg (d.w.). With an increasing amount of buckwheat, the rutin content in bread increased as well (**Figure 7**).

To confirm the positive effects of daily consumption of bread enriched by buckwheat, the clinical study in a group of volunteers was realised. The bread enriched by 30% of buckwheat (from 34.7 mg/kg to 38.2 mg/kg rutin content [d.w.]) was prepared and consumed daily by a group of research volunteers during a period of 4 weeks. After this time period the selected parameters in blood, as well as anthropometric parameters, were evaluated. Three intravenous blood samples were taken: before the clinical study, immediately after it (after 4 weeks of consuming enriched bread) and after another 4 weeks. The consumption was accompanied by changes in blood biochemical parameters (cholesterol level, LDL, HDL, triglycerides), selected elements (Ca, Mg, Fe), creatinine, urea, chloride, glucose and total antioxidant status. The daily consumption of buckwheat enriched bread during the clinical study by volunteers led to a significant increase of the iron level in the blood and a significant decrease of calcium and magnesium. The significant decrease of the HDL cholesterol level was surprising as well as not desirable [64–66]. On the other hand, the expected and welcome decrease of the total cholesterol was statistically insignificant (**Figure 8**). Among the positive changes, there was a significant decrease in the triglyceride and creatinine level and an insignificant decrease in the chloride and urea level.

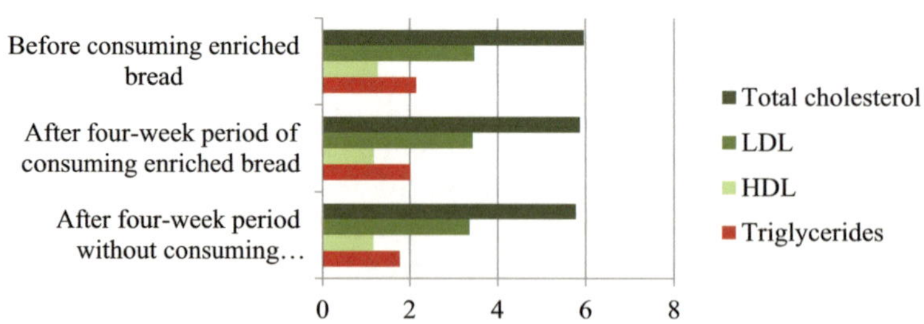

Figure 8.
Total cholesterol, low-density lipoprotein (LDL), high-density lipoprotein (HLD) cholesterol and triglycerides levels (mmol/l) in the blood of volunteers.

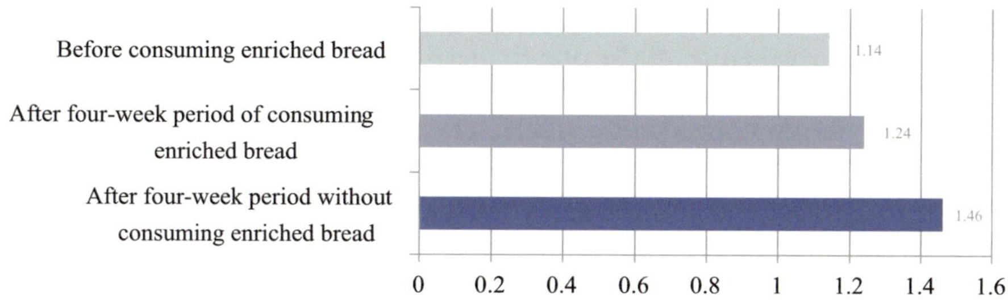

Figure 9.
Total antioxidant status (mmol/l) in volunteers blood.

The powerful antioxidant activity of flavonoids in buckwheat suggests that these compounds could play a protective role in oxidative stress-mediated diseases [29, 67]. The results confirmed the increase of the total antioxidant status (TAS) in consumers eating buckwheat enriched bread (**Figure 9**). The most significant increase in comparison to the initial state was found with research volunteers with an initially low TAS, the increase reached nearly 40%. The highest TAS level (initially as well as finally) was found with younger research volunteers between 18 and 34 years old, the lowest with people between 35 and 54 years old. These data suggested that buckwheat was a significant antioxidant as TAS in human plasma and that the increased TAS level through doses of buckwheat bread could be useful as a free radical scavenger. It appeared that the TAS of the plasma of the volunteers who consumed buckwheat enriched bread daily during the period of 4 weeks was significantly higher than before its consumption. It was interesting to note that 4 weeks after the end of the consumption of buckwheat bread, a further increase in TAS was confirmed, and thus the body's ability to respond with a delay. Based on the findings, we assume that it is not possible to expect an immediate improvement in the required parameters characterising the body's health by changing the diet. It takes longer, and vice versa, after a certain diet, its positive effects persist for a long time.

In general, it can be concluded that the regular consumption of buckwheat enriched bread brings nutritional benefits to the consumers. Long-term consumption can have a protective effect, thanks to the numerous nutraceutical compounds of buckwheat. It is not realistic, though, to expect that the consumption of buckwheat bread would solve the health problems related to an unhealthy lifestyle and bad eating habits in general.

Based on the obtained results we can conclude that the buckwheat addition worsens the technological parameters of the blends used for the baking test. The rheological properties of the dough changed when the amount of buckwheat in the blend was increased. It means that the increased addition of buckwheat caused a lower dough resistance and instability during kneading. The baking test confirmed this, too. The loaves prepared with an addition of buckwheat were evaluated to be of lesser quality. The overall acceptability rating led to the conclusion that bread could be baked with satisfactory results after addition of buckwheat up to 30%.

In addition to the above described and recommended method of application of buckwheat to bread, in mixtures with wheat or rye flour, buckwheat is considered a very important ingredient for gluten-free formulations too [68]. Within the technologies of their production, when wheat flour does not form any portion in the composite flour, the preparation of the dough is more demanding, especially for the production of bread and pastries with the required volume and porosity [69]. The increase of buckwheat flour in standard gluten-free flours results in an increased dough development time and a weakening of the protein network, and a decrease of the starch retrogradation degree. This indicates that the addition of buckwheat flour to gluten-free bread or other bakery products could lead to a product with improved anti-staling properties [70].

The diet based on gluten-free products is characterised by a low content of some nutritional components such as proteins and minerals, as well as non-nutritional components like dietary fibre. Especially for these reasons, buckwheat seeds are an excellent raw material. For example, the addition of 40% of buckwheat flour in standard gluten-free flour produced bread with high overall quality. Buckwheat flour as a natural source of minerals and antioxidant activity, and also as a structure-forming source and improving the sensory quality, can be used for the preparation of buckwheat enhanced gluten-free breads [71].

Buckwheat can therefore be considered, especially thanks to its nutritional benefits, as a raw material suitable as a supplement in a certain amount for the production of classic bread made from wheat flour, but also for the production of gluten-free bread.

4.2 Application of common buckwheat to pasta

Besides using the buckwheat in the production of bread and pastries, as described in the previous sub-section, buckwheat flour can be processed into various non-bakery products such as noodles or pasta. Noodles made from buckwheat flour-water dough are popular in some regions including Japan, where the traditional methods of preparing buckwheat noodles generally consist of six successive processes *(mizu-mawashi, kukuri, kiku-neri, nobashi, tatami, houchhou)*. Apart from the type of flour used, the particle size of flour for noodles and pasta is also important since the data show that a positive correlation between the average diameter of buckwheat flour particles and the maximum water absorption capacity was found. It means that buckwheat flour with a larger particle size can exhibits a higher water absorption capacity than buckwheat flour with smaller particle size [72].

Pasta belongs to the most favourite dishes, especially for young people. The consumption of pasta has a long-term upward trend, so it is important to pay a lot of attention to its production and to improve its nutritional and sensory quality. In particular, pasta belongs to high-carbohydrate foods, which are an important source of energy. It is easily digestible and can be fortified with nutritionally interesting substances, as the easy preparation of pasta enables it. An important feature of pasta is its high degree of flexibility regarding its possible enrichment by different raw materials. If it is specifically designed from certain types of raw materials, it can be consumed as a safe food for certain types of diseases, such as celiac disease [73]. Given that pasta is not a porosity product with a need for gas retention (as with bread), but is a product prepared by cold extrusion, it is possible to use naturally gluten-free raw materials for their production.

Technologically, the most suitable raw material for the production of pasta is semolina, which is flour made from durum wheat (*Triticum durum* L.) and flour from common wheat (*Triticum aestivum* L.).

The experimental pasta was produced in a Fimar MPF 25 low-pressure extruder, in which 25–35% water, eggs, and salt were added to the flour. The formed dense dough was mixed for 15 min, then extruded through an extruder stamper and cut. In addition to the production of traditional pasta, the attention was focused on the preparation of products with a higher nutritional potential. Samples of semolina and common wheat flour were prepared as controls, to be compared with the gluten-free pasta from buckwheat wholegrain flour and composite flour from buckwheat flour and rice flour in a ratio of 50:50. The pasta was dried to the required moisture (<13%), and the dried pasta was evaluated by the water activity (a_w, Novasina), which is an important indicator of the stability and durability of the products. The water activity values of pasta ranged from 0.538 to 0.552, and it can be stated that it achieved a satisfactory value for this characteristic which is below 0.6. This is a value of an activity corresponding to microbiological stability [19].

From a nutritional point of view, the application of buckwheat has brought into the system a high content of protein (in buckwheat flour 18% d.w., Kjeldahl) and minerals (in buckwheat flour 2.6% d.w., ash content), which was also transferred to pasta. Compared to the control products, the protein and minerals content was considerably higher, as documented in **Figure 10**.

The acidity of flours is indicated by the amount of acidic substances, which are represented by the presence of free fatty acids (products of hydrolytic fats breakdown), phosphates (formed by the breakdown of organic phosphorus compounds such as phytin, phospholipids), and protein hydrolysis products. A higher acidity was found in highly ground and wholemeal flours and groats, and the content of acidic substances also increased with the length of their storage [3]. The acid value of pasta from common wheat was very low (15 mmol/kg) and predicted less pronounced pasta. A high acidity was found in pasta from wholegrain buckwheat, and from a mixture of buckwheat and rice flour, since wholegrain buckwheat flour was used.

Based on the evaluation of the pasta experiment, a comparable level of the ability to be boiled was found. The cooking time of pasta, the binding of the water which is absorbed during cooking, the swelling, which expresses the increase in the volume of cooked pasta and sediment, or cooking losses, confirmed satisfactory values of these parameters in all samples of the experimental pasta. Compared to the control pasta, only the sediment values (cooking losses) of the whole grain buckwheat flour pasta were 100% higher. The sensory evaluation of raw pasta monitored its general appearance, surface properties, flexibility, and strength. After cooking, the sensory profile monitored colour, aroma, taste, stickiness, and general impression. After evaluating the pasta's sensory quality before and after cooking, it can be concluded that the pasta's sensory profile was at a comparable level with the control products. However, the raw and cooked pasta from semolina and common wheat flour had the highest score (**Figure 11**).

Pasta from composite flours was prepared as well. In these flours, whole grain buckwheat flour was added to common wheat flour in amounts of 10, 20, 30, 40, and 50%. All additions increased the content of minerals and proteins in proportion to the

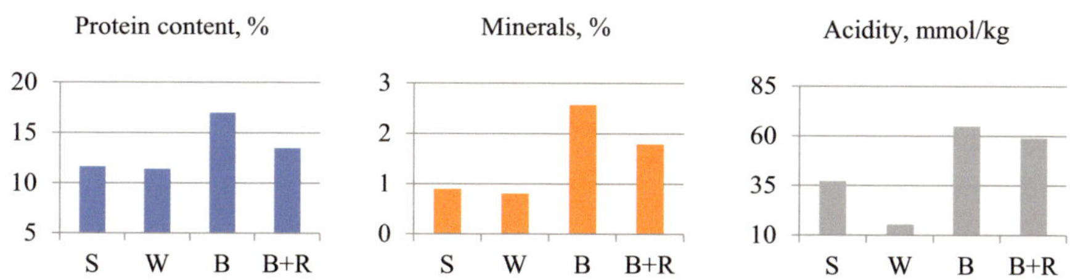

Figure 10.
Graphic overview of protein content, minerals content, and titrable acidity in control pasta and in gluten-free pasta with buckwheat. S-semolina, W-common wheat flour, B-buckwheat wholegrain flour 100%, B + R-buckwheat whole flour + rice flour 50:50.

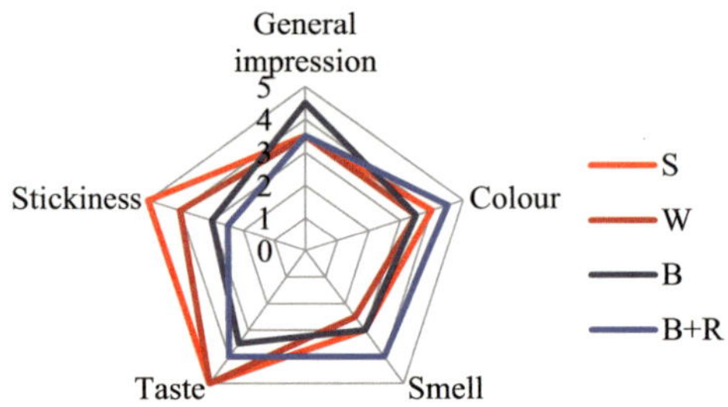

Figure 11.
Sensory evaluation of pasta after cooking. S-semolina, W-common wheat flour, B-buckwheat wholegrain flour 100%, B + R-buckwheat whole flour + rice flour 50:50. 0-the worst evaluation, 5-the best evaluation.

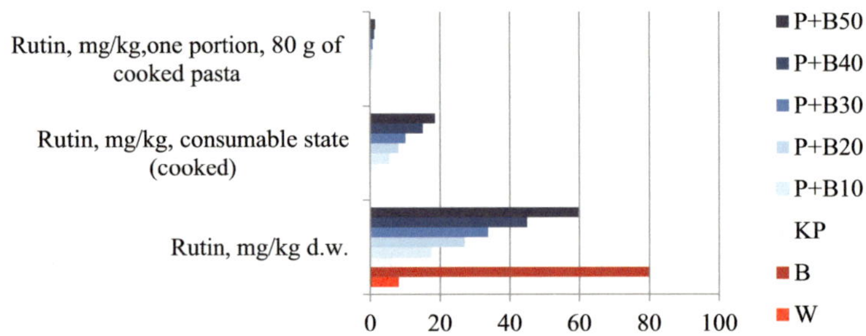

Figure 12.
Rutin content in pasta (dry, after cooking and in one consumable portion).

amount added. What was even more important, however, was the increasing content of rutin in buckwheat-enriched pasta (**Figure 12**), and its content in cooked pasta in the consumable state and per serving (80 g of cooked pasta) [72].

Based on our findings, we can conclude that pasta from buckwheat has excellent technological, nutritional, and sensory qualities.

5. Conclusions

This chapter describes the benefits and possible risks, of the inclusion of common buckwheat into the diet. Buckwheat seeds have a very attractive composition. In addition to essential nutrients, which are a source of energy and have other physiological functions, they also contain biologically active compounds that support the good health of consumers. For food production, the usable part of buckwheat is buckwheat achene, which is dehulled. The focus is on food products of daily consumption (bread and pasta) prepared with a portion of buckwheat flour of 10–50%.

The application of common buckwheat to bread as food consumed on a daily basis and generally very popular has proven to be a very convenient way of making bread more nutritionally attractive. Analyses using rheological and fermentographic methods revealed the following modes of behaviour of the dough with the addition of buckwheat flour:

- the influence of buckwheat added to composite flours on the properties evaluated by a farinograph was significant. While increasing the portion of buckwheat, the dough consistency (in comparison to wheat flour) decreased, the dough became weaker and the resistance against the farinograph blades was lower,

- when preparing doughs with non-bakery raw materials, it is necessary to consider, verify, and set the optimal kneading mode,

- the gas volume and retention volume with an addition of 30% of buckwheat flour (an acceptable amount of the addition) were comparable to the control sample from wheat flour, which provided a precondition for a reasonable volume of the final product—bread,

- based on a baking experiment we can state that increasing the buckwheat amount in blends with wheat flour caused the decrease of important parameters such as loaf volume, specific loaf volume, and volume efficiency,

- the overall acceptability of the breads in a sensory evaluation decreased with the amount of buckwheat flour addition, but ≤30% buckwheat flour gave acceptable results,

- from the overall acceptability rating, it was concluded that bread with additions of 10%, 20%, and 30% of buckwheat could be baked with satisfactory results,

- in general, it can be concluded that the regular consumption of buckwheat enriched bread brings nutritional benefits to the consumers.

The application of common buckwheat to pasta can play an important role given that the consumption of pasta has a long-term upward trend in the population. An important feature of pasta is its high degree of flexibility regarding its possible enrichment by different raw materials. Analyses and evaluations of pasta prepared with an addition of buckwheat flour to wheat flour confirmed that:

- from a nutritional point of view, the application of buckwheat brought into the system a high content of protein and minerals, which was also transferred to pasta,

- the cooking time of pasta, the binding of the water which is absorbed during cooking, the swelling, which expresses the increase in the volume of cooked pasta and sediment, or cooking losses, confirmed satisfactory values of these parameters in all samples of the experimental pasta,

- after evaluating the pasta's sensory quality before and after cooking, it can be concluded that the pasta's sensory profile was at a comparable level with the control products,

- all additions increased the content of rutin in buckwheat-enriched pasta proportionally to the amount of the addition.

Based on the findings and results of the analyses, common buckwheat can be recommended as an ingredient of basic carbohydrate foods such as bread or pasta.

Acknowledgements

This study was supported by the grant VEGA 1/0113/21 "Marginal plant sources of biologically active substances with a possibility of its application in food products".

Author details

Tatiana Bojňanská*, Alena Vollmannová, Judita Lidiková and Janette Musilová
Slovak University of Agriculture in Nitra, Slovak Republic

*Address all correspondence to: tatiana.bojnanska@uniag.sk

References

[1] Zhou M, Tang Y, Deng X, Ruan C, Kreft I, Tang Y, et al. Overview of buckwheat resources in the world. In: Zhou M, Kreft I, Suvorova G, Tang Y, Woo SH, editors. Buckwheat Germplasm in the World. 1st ed. London, United Kingdom: Academic Press; 2018. pp. 1-7. DOI: 10.1016/B978-0-12-811006-500001-X

[2] Davidson A. The Oxford Companion to Food. 1st ed. Oxford, United Kingdom: Oxford University Press; 1999. p. 892. ISBN 0-19-211579-0

[3] Bojňanská T, Muchová Z, Frančáková H, Urminská D, Mendelová A, Mareček J, et al. Hodnotenie surovín a potravín rastlinného pôvodu (Evaluation of Raw Materials and Foods of Plant Origin). 1st ed. Nitra: Slovak University of Agriculture; 2013. 335 p. ISBN 978-80-552-1086-5

[4] Kováč L, Jakubová J. Teplomilné plodiny na ťažkých pôdach a ekonomika ich pestovania (Thermophilic Crops on Heavy Soils and the Economics of Their Cultivation). 1st ed. Lužianky: National Agricultural and Food Center; 2017. p. 72. ISBN 978-80-971644-7-8

[5] Yilmaz HO, Ayhan NY, Meriç CS. Buckwheat: A useful food and its effects on human health. Current Nutrition & Food Science. 2020;**16**:29-34. DOI: 10.2174/1573401314666180910140021

[6] Huda MN, Lua S, Jahan T, Ding M, Jha R, Zhang K, et al. Treasure from garden: Bioactive compounds of buckwheat. Food Chemistry. 2021;**335**: 127653. DOI: 10.1016/j.foodchem.2020.127653

[7] Zhu F. Buckwheat proteins and peptides: Biological functions and food applications. Trends in Food Science & Technology. 2021;**110**:155-140. DOI: 10.1016/j.tifs.2021.01.081

[8] Krkošková B, Mrázova Z. Prophylactic components of buckwheat. Food Research International. 2005;**38**:561-568. DOI: 10.1016/j.foodres.2004.11.009

[9] Wijngaard HH, Arendt EK. Buckwheat. Cereal Chemistry. 2006;**83**(4):391-401. DOI: 10.1094/ CC-83-0391

[10] Petr J, Michalík I, Tlaskalová H, Capouchová I, Faměra O, Urminská D, et al. Extention of the spectra of plant products for the diet in coeliac disease. Czech Journal of Food Science. 2003;**21**(2):59-70

[11] Radovic RS, Maksimovic RV, Brkljacic MJ, Varkonji Gasic IE, Savic PA. 2S albumin from buckwheat (*Fagopyrum esculentum*) seeds. Journal of Agricultural and Food Chemistry. 1999;**47**:1467-1470. DOI: 10.1021/jf980778s

[12] Skrabanja V, Kreft I. Resistant starch formation following autoclaving of buckwheat (*Fagopyrum esculentum* Moench) groats. An in vitro study. Journal of Agricultural and Food Chemistry. 1998;**46**:2020-2023. DOI: 10.1021/jf970756q

[13] Dziedzic K, Górecka D, Kucharska M, Przybylska B. Influence of technological process during buckwheat groats production on dietary fibre content and sorption of bile acids. Food Research International. 2012;**47**:279-283. DOI: 10.1016/j.foodres.2011.07.020

[14] Soliman GA. Dietary fiber, atherosclerosis, and cardiovascular disease. Nutrients. 2019;**11**:1155. DOI: 10.3390/nu11051155

[15] Vojtíšková P, Švec P, Kubáň V, Krejzová E, Bittová M, Kráčmar S, et al. Chemical composition of buckwheat

plant parts and selected buckwheat products. Potravinárstvo (Slovak Journal of Food Sciences). 2014;**8**:247-253. DOI: 10.5219/385

[16] Gulpinar AR, Orhan IE, Kan A, Seno FS, Celik SA, Kartal M. Estimation of in vitro neuroprotective properties and quantification of rutin and fatty acids in buckwheat (*Fagopyrum esculentum* Moench) cultivated in Turkey. Food Research International. 2012;**46**:536-543. DOI: 10.1016/j.foodres.2011.08.011

[17] Skrabanja V, Kreft I, Golob T, Modic M, Ikeda S, Kiyokazu I, et al. Nutrient content in buckwheat milling fractions. Cereal Chemistry. 2004;**81**:172-176. DOI: 10.1094/CCHEM.2004.81.2.172

[18] Pongrac P, Vogel-Mikuš K, Potisek M, Kovačec E, Budič B, Kump P, et al. Mineral and trace element composition and importance for nutritional value of buckwheat grain, groats, and sprouts. In: Zhou M, Kreft I, Woo SH, Chrungoo N, Wieslander G, editors. Molecular Breeding and Nutritional Aspects of Buckwheat. London, United Kingdom: Academic Press; 2016. pp. 261-271. DOI: 10.1016/B978-0-12-803692-1.00020-1

[19] Velíšek J, Hajšlová J. Chemie potravin I (Food chemistry I). 3rd ed. Tábor: OSIS—Ing.Václav Šedivý; 2009. p. 602. ISBN 978-80-86659-15-2

[20] Bystrická J, Vollmannová A, Čičová I, Bojňanská T, Margitanová E. Variability of bioactive compounds in buckwheat (*Fagopyrum esculentum* Moench.). In: Proceeding of the Crop Science for Food Security, Bioenergy and Sustainability (3rd IFSDAA International Seminar), Society for Sustainable Agriculture and Resource Management. Szeged, Hungary; 1-3 June 2010. p. 109

[21] Bystrická J, Vollmannová A, Kupecsek A, Musilová J, Poláková Z, Čičová I, et al. Bioactive compounds in different plant parts of various buckwheat (*Fagopyrum esculentum* Moench.) cultivars. Cereal research communications. 2011;**39**(3):436-444. DOI: 10.1556/CRC.39.2011.3.13

[22] Vollmannová A, Bojňanská T, Urminská D, Čičová I. Translocation of phenolics and rutin in different anatomical plant parts of buckwheat and amaranth. In: Book of Abstracts and Posters of the 12th International Scientific Conference Biotechnology and Quality of Raw Materials and Foodstuffs; 16-18 May, 2017. Nitra: Slovak University of Agriculture; 2017. p. 129. ISBN 978-80-552-1669-0

[23] Borovaya SA, Klykov AG. Some aspects of flavonoid biosynthesis and accumulation in buckwheat plants: Review. Plant Biotechnology Reports. 2020;**14**:213-225. DOI: 10.1007/s11816-020-00614-9

[24] Vollmannová A, Musilová J, Lidiková J, Árvay J, Šnirc M, Tóth T, et al. Concentrations of phenolic acids are differently genetically determined in leaves, flowers, and grain of common buckwheat (*Fagopyrum esculentum* Moench). Plants. 2021;**10**:1142. DOI: 10.3390/plants10061142

[25] Bystrická J, Musilová J, Vollmannová A, Lachman J, Kavalcová P. Changes of Polyphenolic Substances in the Anatomical Parts of Buckwheat (*Fagopyrum esculentum* Moench) during Its Growth Phases. Food. 2014;**3**:558-568. DOI: 10.3390/foods3040558

[26] Vollmannová A, Margitanová E, Tóth T, Urminská D, Bojňanská T. Cultivar influence on total polyphenol and rutin contents and total antoxidant capacity in buckwheat, amaranth and quinoa seeds. In: Proceeding of the Chemical Reactions in Food VII; 14-16 November 2012. Praha: Institute of

Chemical Technology; 2012. p. 107. ISBN 978-80-7080-836-8

[27] Kreft I, Fabjan N, Yasumoto K. Rutin content in buckwheat (*Fagopyrum esculentum* Moench.) food materials and products. Food Chemistry. 2006;**98**:508-512. DOI: 10.1016/j.foodchem.2005.05.081

[28] Steadman KJ, Burgoon MS, Lewis BA, Edwardson SE, Obendorf RL. Minerals, phytic acid, tannin and rutin in buckwheat seed milling fractions. Journal of the Science of Food and Agriculture. 2001;**81**:1094-1100. DOI: 10.1002/jsfa.914

[29] Bojňanská T, Fikselová M. Antioxidačný účinok a obsah rutínu v pšeničných chleboch s rozličným prídavkom pohánky (antioxidant effect and rutin content in wheat breads with various buckwheat additions). In: Proceedings of the 1st Annual Scientific Conference with International Participation Antioxidants 2009; 6 May 2009. Nitra: Slovak University of Agriculture; 2009. pp. 19-25. ISBN 978-80-552-0209-9

[30] Holasova M, Fiedlerova H, Smrcinova H, Orsak M, Lachman J, Vavreinova S. Buckwheat—the source of antioxidant activity in functional foods. Food Research International. 2002;**35**:207-211. DOI: 10.1016/A0963-9969(01)00185-5

[31] Musilová J, Lachman J, Bystrická J, Vollmannová A, Čičová I, Timoracká M. Cultivar and growth phases—the factors affecting antioxidant activity of buckwheat (*Fagopyrum esculentum* Moench). Acta Agriculturae Slovenica. 2013;**101**(2):201-208. DOI: 10.2478/acas-2013-0016

[32] Hon Z, Patočka J. Pojanka jako funkční potravina (buckwheat as a functional food). Kontakt. 2008;**10**(1):229-231. DOI: 10.32725/kont.2008.032

[33] Kim J, Hwang KT. Fagopyrins in different parts of common buckwheat (*Fagopyrum esculentum*) and Tartary buckwheat (*F. tataricum*) during growth. Journal of Food Composition and Analysis. 2020;**86**:103354. DOI: 10.1016/j.jfca.2019.103354

[34] Matsumoto R, Fujino K, Nagata Y, Hashiguchi S, Ito Y, Aihara Y, et al. Molecular characterization of a 10-kDa buckwheat molecule reactive to allergic patients´ IgE. Allergy. 2004;**59**(5):533-538. DOI: 10.1046/j.1398-9995.2003.00412.x

[35] Heffler E, Pizzimenti S, Badiu I, Guida G, Rolla G. Buckwheat allergy: An emerging clinical problem in Europe. Allergy & Therapy. 2014;**2**(5):168. DOI: 10.4172/2155-6121.100016

[36] Dietrich-Szostak D, Oleszek W. Effect of processing on the flavonoid content in buckwheat (*Fagpyrum esculentum* Moench) grain. Journal of Agricultural and Food Chemistry. 1999;**47**:4384-4387. DOI: 10.1021/jf990121m

[37] Bulletin of the Ministry of Health of the Slovak Republic. 63/4-5. June 19, 2015

[38] Valavanidis A. Bread, Oldest Man-made Staple Food in Human Diet Bread Intake Is Integral to Good Health and Whole Grain Cereals Beneficial against Chronic Diseases [Internet]. 2018. Available from: www.chem-tox-ecotox.org/ScientificReviews [Accessed: November 15, 2018]

[39] Bojňanská T, Musilová J, Vollmannová A. Effects of adding legume flours on the rheological and breadmaking properties of dough.

Food. 2021;**10**:1087. DOI: 10.3390/foods10051087

[40] Bojňanská T, Urminská D. Enriched bread—A source of biologically active components in nutrition. In: The Abstract Book. Vitamins 2007: Nutrition and Diagnostic; Prague Czech Republic; 19-21 September 2007; Pardubice: Univerzita Pardubice. 2007. p. 123. ISBN 978-80-7194-937-4

[41] Bojňanská T, Urminská D. Buckwheat (*Fagopyrum esculentum* Moench.) a source of biologically active components bread. Chem. 2007;**3**(1):218-219. ISSN 1336-7242

[42] Bojňanská T, Frančáková H, Gažar R. Vplyv prídavku pohánky na technologickú a nutričnú kvalitu chleba (Influence of buckwheat addition on technological and nutritional quality of bread). Acta fytotechnica et zootechnica. 2009;**12**:57-63. ISSN 1335-258X

[43] Bojňanská T, Frančáková H, Chlebo P, Gažar R. Možnosti využitia pohánky pri výrobe chleba a výhody jeho konzumácie (possibilities of using buckwheat in the production of bread and the benefits of its consumption). Potravinárstvo (Slovak Journal of Food Sciences). 2010;**4**(1):8-12. ISSN 1338-0230. ISSN 1337-0960

[44] Margier M, Georgé S, Hafnaoui N, Remond D, Nowicki M, Du Chaffaut L, et al. Nutritional composition and bioactive content of legumes: Characterization of pulses frequently consumed in france and effect of the cooking method. Nutrients. 2018;**10**:1668. DOI: 10.3390/nu10111668

[45] Torbica A, Belovič M, Tomič J. Novel breads of non-wheat flours. Food Chemistry. 2019;**282**:134-140. DOI: 10.1016/j.foodchem.2018.12.113

[46] Bojňanská T, Ivanišová E, Vollmannová A, Kreft I. Efekt prídavku pohánky na reologické vlastnosti cesta a kvalitu pohánkového chleba (the effect of buckwheat addition on the rheological properties of dough and the quality of buckwheat bread). In: Podpora výskumných aktivít vo VC ABT (Support of Research Activities in RC ABT). 1st ed. Nitra: Slovak University of Agriculture; 2019. pp. 64-74. ISBN 978-80-552-2125-0

[47] Rosell CM, Santos E, Collar C. Physical characterization of fiber-enriched bread doughs by dual mixing and temperature constraint using the Mixolab®. European Food Research and Technology. 2010;**231**:535-544. DOI: 10.1007/s00217-010-1310-y

[48] Hadnađev TD, Torbica A, Hadnađev M. Rheological properties of wheat flour substitutes/alternative crops assessed by Mixolab. Procedia Food Science. 2011;**1**:328-334. DOI: 10.1016/j.profoo.2011.09.051

[49] Gažar R, Bojňanská T. Vplyv prídavku pohánky na reologické vlastnosti pšeničného cesta a kvalitu chleba (Influence of buckwheat addition on the rheological properties of wheat dough and bread quality). In: Proceedings of the II. Scientific Conference of Doctoral Students: With International Participation on the Occasion of the 1st Year of the VEDA—EDUCATION—PRACTICE Fair and the European Science Week; Nitra; 16 November 2007. Nitra: Slovak University of Agriculture; 2007. pp. 190-193. ISBN 978-80-8069-959-8

[50] Bojňanská T, Urminská D, Bennár M, Gažar R. Influence of natural additives on rheological properties of wheat dough. In: Proceedings of the FoodInnova: International Conference on Food Inovation; Valencia, Spain; 25-29 October 2010. Vol. 120. Valencia:

Universitat Politecnica de Valencia; 2010. pp. 1-4. ISBN 978-84-693-5010-2

[51] Wieser H. Chemistry of gluten proteins. Food Microbiology. 2007;**24**:115-119. DOI: 10.1016/j.fm.2006.07.004

[52] Bojňanská T, Tokár M, Gažar R. Pharinographic characteristics of wheat douch with natural additives. Journal of Food Physics. 2010;**23**:9-12. ISSN 1416-3365

[53] Lazaridou A, Duta D, Papageorgiou M, Belc N, Biliaderis CG. Effects of hydrocolloids on dough rheology and bread quality parameters in gluten-free formulations. Journal of Food Engineering. 2007;**79**:1033-1047. DOI: 10.16/j.jfoodeng.2006.03.032

[54] Bojňanská T, Šmitalová J, Vollmannová A, Ivanišová E. Addition of non-bakery raw materials and their influence on the properties of dough and bakery products. In: Proceedings of the 4rd International Scientific—Practical Conference Innovative Technologies in Bakery Production; 17 November 2020. Kyiv, Ukraine: National University of Food Technologies; 2020. pp. 17-22. ISBN UDK 664.6

[55] Roccia P, Ribotta PD, Pérez GT, León AE. Influence of soy protein on rheological properties and water retention capacity of wheat gluten. LWT—Food Science and Technology. 2009;**42**:358-362. DOI: 10.1016/j.lwt.2008.03.002

[56] Bojňanská T, Šmitalová J. The influence of additional fluors on the retention ability of dough and the technological quality of bakery products. Potravinárstvo (Slovak Journal of Food Sciences). 2015;**9**(1):242-246. DOI: 10.5219/468

[57] Bojňanská T, Vollmannová A, Musilová J, Urminská D, Habánová M. Non-bakery raw materials with nutritional potential and their influence on the rheofermentographic properties of dough. In: Proceedings of the CzechFoodChem2021; online; 24-26 May 2021. Czech Republic: Food Research Institute Prague; 2021. p. 41-46. ISBN 978-80-7592-102-4

[58] Rosell CM, Collar C, Haros M. Assessment of hydrocolloid effects on the thermo-mechanical properties of wheat using the Mixolab. Food Hydrocolloids. 2007;**21**:452-462. DOI: 10.1016/j.foodhyd.2006.05.004

[59] Bonafaccia G, Marocchini M, Kreft I. Composition and technological properties of the flour and bran from common and tartary buckwheat. Food Chemistry. 2003;**80**:9-15. DOI: 10.1016/S0308-8146(02)00228-5

[60] Cauvain SP, editor. Bread making. In: Improving Quality. 1st ed. Cambridge: Woodhead Publishing Ltd; 2003. 589 p. ISBN 1 85573 553 9

[61] Cauvain SP, Young LS. Technology of Breadmaking. 2nd ed. New York, USA: Springer Science+Business Media; 2007. p. 397. ISBN 978-0-387-38563-1

[62] Bojňanská T, Urminská D. Influence of natural additives on protein complex of bread. Potravinárstvo (Slovak Journal of Food Sciences). 2010;**4**(4):1-5. DOI: 10.5219/77

[63] Bojňanská T, Horna A, Habánová M. Buckwheat (*Fagopyrum esculentum* Moench.)—A source of rutin in human nutrition. In: Proceedings of the Vitamins 2008—Nutrition and Diagnostics: 8th International Conference; 9-11 September 2008. Zlín. Zlín, Czech Republic: Univerzita Tomáše Bati; 2008. pp. 44-45. ISBN 978-80-7318-708-8

[64] Bojňanská T, Chlebo P, Habánová M, Habán M. Effect of rutin in consumed bread on blood parameters of volunteers. Acta fytotechnica et zootechnica. 2011;**14**:36-39. ISSN 1335-258X. Available from: http://www.slpk.sk/acta/docs/2011/afz-si2011/afzsi2011-36-39.pdf

[65] Bojňanská T, Chlebo P, Horna A, Gažar R. Buckwheat enrichment bread production and its nutrition benefits. European Journal of Plant Science and Biotechnology, Global Science Books. 2009;**3**(1):49-55. ISSN 1752-3842. ISBN 978-4-903313-42-9

[66] Bojňanská T, Chlebo P, Urminská D, Gažar R. Buckwheat enriched bread production and its nutritional benefits. Annals of Nutrition & Metabolism. 2013;**63**(1):1718. ISSN 0250-6807

[67] Bojňanská T, Frančáková H, Chlebo P, Vollmannová A. Rutin content in buckwheat enriched bread and influence of its consumption on plasma total antioxidant status. Czech Journal of Food Science. 2009;**27**:S236-S240. DOI: 10.17221/967-CJFS

[68] Giménez Bastida JA, Zielinski H. Buckwheat as a functional food and its effects on health. Journal of Agricultural and Food Chemistry. 2015;**63**(36):7896-7913. DOI: 10.1021/acj.jafc.5b02498

[69] Dvořáková P, Burešová I, Kráčmar S. Buckwhet as a gluten-free cereal in combination with maize flour. Journal of Microbiology, Biotechnology and Food Sciences. 2012;**1**:897-907

[70] Torbica A, Hadnađev M, Dapčević T. Rheological, textural and sensory properties of gluten-free bread formulations based on rice and buckwheat flour. Food Hydrocolloids. 2010;**24**:626-632. DOI: 10.1016/j.foodhyd.2010.03.004

[71] Wronkowska M, Zielinska D, Szawara-Nowak D, Troszynska A, Soral-Smietana M. Antioxidative and reducing capacity, macroelements content and sensorial properties of buckwheat-enhanced gluten-free bread. Food Science & Technology. 2010;**45**:1993-2000. DOI: 10.1111/j.1365-2621.2010.02375.x

[72] Asami Y, Yamashita Y, Oka T, Terao T, Ito S, Ikeda S, et al. Analysis of traditional preparation methods of buckwheat noodles in Japan. Fagopyrum. 2018;**35**:19-27. DOI: 10.3986/fag0003

[73] Bojňanská T, Muchová Z. The technological and nutritional quality of enriched non-yeast cereal products. In: Proceeding of the Security and Quality of Raw Materials and Foods Conference; 9 November 2006. Nitra: Slovak University of Agriculture; 2006. pp. 45-49. ISBN 80-8069-767-1

Chapter 3

Proteins from Pseudocereal Grains

Asli Can Karaca

Abstract

Seeds such as quinoa, amaranth, chia, and teff are considered as potential sources of plant-based proteins for human consumption. Proteins isolated from pseudocereal grains have the potential to serve as nutritious alternatives to animal-based proteins for various food applications. Quinoa, amaranth, and chia proteins are among the most extensively studied pseudocereal proteins for the characterization of structural, physicochemical, and functional properties. This chapter will review the recent studies on composition, structural characteristics, physicochemical and functional properties of proteins isolated from pseudocereal grains, will discuss several modifications applied for improvement of functional properties and some potential end-product applications.

Keywords: pseudocereal protein, functional properties, physicochemical properties, chia, quinoa, amaranth

1. Introduction

Pseudocereal grains are considered as good sources of protein with a balanced amino acid profile. Proteins from pseudocereal grains have recently gained increasing popularity due to their nutritional, functional, and biological properties. Proteins from quinoa, amaranth, and chia are among the most extensively studied pseudocereal proteins in terms of characterization of physicochemical, functional, and biological properties. The functionality of proteins from other less known pseudocereals, such as kiwicha and cañihua, still remains to be explored. Although proteins from pseudocereal grains are indicated to show good functionality, some processes may be required to modify the structure and improve the functionality of pseudocereal proteins. Structural and functional properties of various pseudocereal proteins are recently reviewed [1–3]. This chapter presents an overview of the structural and functional properties of pseudocereal proteins, the effects of methods used for protein extraction and fractionation on protein functionality, and several methods applied for modification of structure and optimizing the functionality of pseudocereal proteins.

2. Quinoa protein

Quinoa (*Chenopodium quinoa* Willd) contains ~13–16% protein with major fractions of albumins (29–50%) and globulins (7–37%) classified based on the extraction methodology [2, 4–6]. Structural and functional properties of quinoa protein were recently reviewed by Dakhili et al. [2]. Quinoa seed protein is reported to contain a balanced essential amino acid profile, with relatively higher amounts of lysine and methionine compared to cereals and legumes [5]. Physicochemical and functional properties of quinoa protein were investigated in recent studies to elucidate its potential for utilization as an ingredient in various food applications. It has been indicated that the method used for protein extraction has a significant effect on the composition and functionality of quinoa protein [2]. Moreover, inert physical barriers in the seed are indicated to hinder a significant portion of protein in quinoa from being extracted [6]. Van de Vondel et al. [6] recently investigated heat-induced protein denaturation and aggregation during protein extraction from quinoa using denaturing agent sodium dodecyl sulfate (SDS) and reducing agent dithiothreitol (DTT) with an aim to maximize extraction yield. The maximum protein extraction yield obtained using SDS, DTT, and/or various pretreatments was reported to be 82%, which indicated that physical barriers hinder the extraction of ~20–25% of the protein in quinoa [6].

Various physical, chemical, and biological modification methods are applied to pseudocereal proteins to improve functionality. Enzymatic hydrolysis is a commonly applied strategy to improve not only the functional but also the bioactive properties of plant-based proteins. Guo et al. [7] recently reviewed the biological activities of quinoa protein hydrolysate and peptides. In a recent study, Daliri et al. [8] applied enzymatic hydrolysis to quinoa protein concentrate with pancreatin and investigated the changes in emulsifying, foaming, and antioxidant properties. Quinoa protein concentrate was obtained from defatted quinoa flour with alkaline extraction followed by the isoelectric precipitation method. Hydrolysis with pancreatin at 40°C for 180 min was reported to result in the highest degree of hydrolysis (~19%). Fourier-transform infrared spectroscopy analysis revealed that different functional groups, such as free regions of hydroxylic amino acids, aromatic amino acids, and free amino groups, originated in the hydrolysate due to the hydrolyzing action of pancreatin. The obtained hydrolysate was reported to show better antioxidant properties in terms of 2,2-diphenyl-1-picrylhydrazyl free radical scavenging activity. Solubility, emulsifying and foaming activities of the hydrolysate were found to be higher than that of the native protein. On the other hand, the native protein showed better emulsion and foam stabilizing properties [8].

Maillard reaction is used as a tool to modify structural properties and improve the functionality and biological activity of proteins. In a recent study, Teng et al. [9] investigated the effect of glycosylation with xylose on the structural and functional properties of quinoa protein. Quinoa protein isolate (96% protein) was obtained from defatted quinoa flour with alkaline extraction followed by an isoelectric precipitation method. Glycosylation via Maillard reaction was performed by mixing quinoa protein isolate with mannose or xylose with varying proportions in phosphate buffer and heating at 60°C for 4 h. The optimum ratio of quinoa protein to monosaccharide was determined to be 2:1 based on the degree of grafting and browning index analyses. The electrophoretic profile of samples revealed that glycosylation had significant effects on the depolymerization and remodeling of molecular aggregates of quinoa protein. The specific surface area and absorption capacity of quinoa protein were indicated to increase after glycosylation. Solubility, water and fat absorption capacities, emulsifying activity, and stability of glycosylated quinoa protein were reported to be significantly higher than that of the native protein. Moreover, anti-inflammatory and anti-proliferative activities of quinoa protein were indicated to increase after the glycosylation reaction [9].

3. Amaranth protein

Amaranth (*Amaranthus* spp.) seeds contain ~13–15% protein with major fractions of albumin, globulin, and glutelin [4, 10]. Tömösközi et al. [11] investigated functional properties of amaranth protein in model systems and used casein and soy protein isolate as reference proteins for comparison. Amaranth protein isolate (80% protein) was obtained from defatted amaranth flour from two different varieties with alkaline extraction followed by the isoelectric precipitation method. Following extraction, amaranth protein isolate was separated into fractions based on the Osborne-type fractionation method. Fractions of albumin, globulin, and glutelin-type alkali-soluble residual proteins were obtained and tested for functionality. The authors observed similarities between protein profiles of soy and amaranth. However, emulsifying and foaming properties of amaranth protein and derived fractions were found to be relatively poor compared to casein and soy protein. Among the amaranth protein fractions, solubilities of albumin and globulin fractions were reported to be significantly higher than that of the residue protein. It was concluded that optimization of protein extraction and enzymatic or chemical modification of protein structure may be required for effective utilization of amaranth protein preparations as food ingredients in various end-product applications [11].

Figueroa-González et al. [12] investigated the effects of pH-shifting and ultrasonication treatments on the structure, physicochemical, and foaming properties of amaranth protein. Amaranth protein isolate (83% protein) was obtained from defatted amaranth flour with alkaline extraction-isoelectric precipitation method. Amaranth protein dispersions were prepared in distilled water (30 mg/mL, pH 7.0) and protein was modified by five different treatments—pH-shifting at pH 2.0 and 12.0, sonication (750 W) for 10 min at an amplitude of 50%, and pH-shifting (at pH 2.0 and 12.0) followed by sonication. After the modification treatments, amaranth protein dispersions were dried at 35°C for 45 h in the oven to avoid protein denaturation. Alkaline pH-shifting followed by sonication was reported to result in a significant decrease in the hydrodynamic diameter of amaranth protein. On the other hand, hydrodynamic diameter of protein was observed to increase after the acidic pH-shifting treatment. The isoelectric point of amaranth protein increased from 4.0 to 4.2 after the alkaline pH-shifting treatment and to 4.5 after the combined alkaline pH-shifting and ultrasound treatments. However, ultrasound treatment alone was reported to decrease the isoelectric point of amaranth protein to 3.5. Alkaline pH-shifting and ultrasound treatments were reported to induce changes in the secondary structure fractions of amaranth protein. Moreover, both pH-shifting treatments and combination of pH-shifting and ultrasound treatments resulted in changes in the sulfhydryl groups and disulfide bonds of amaranth protein. Both pH-shifting treatments were reported to improve the solubility of amaranth protein, where the highest protein solubility was observed in the sample treated with a combination of alkaline pH-shifting and ultrasound. The foaming capacity and stability of amaranth protein were reported to increase significantly after all treatments except for the acidic pH-shifting treatment. Moreover, treatments applied were indicated to improve the *in vitro* digestibility of amaranth protein that was attributed to the modifications in protein structure, which lead to increased accessibility to digestive enzymes [12].

Das et al. [13] investigated the effects of pH treatment and the extraction pH on the physicochemical and functional properties of amaranth protein isolate. Amaranth protein isolate was obtained from defatted amaranth flour with alkaline extraction at different pH values (9.0, 10.0, 11.0, and 12.0) followed by isoelectric precipitation (pH 4.5). Amaranth protein isolates were subjected to pH treatments at pH 3.0–9.0 and tested for functionality. The protein content of amaranth proteins extracted at different pH values changed between 56 and 85%, where the isolate obtained at pH 9.0 showed the highest purity, solubility, and particle size but the lowest yield. The authors reported that maintaining the extraction and treatment pH values at 9.0 resulted in significant improvements in functional properties including solubility, water and oil binding capacities, emulsifying and foaming properties. Extraction and treatment at pH 9.0 were also indicated to result in better thermal properties and improved gelation characteristics. Moreover, emulsifying, foaming, and gelation properties of amaranth protein isolates were reported to be affected by the particle size, wettability, and solubility [13].

Enzymatic modification is recently applied as a useful tool to improve the functionality and biological activity of amaranth protein. Kamal et al. [14] prepared amaranth protein hydrolysates using bromelain, chymotrypsin, and pronase E enzymes at three different hydrolysis durations (2, 4, and 6 h). Bioactive peptides were identified by LC-MS-QToF analysis. Amaranth protein hydrolysates were reported to contain bioactive peptides with inhibitory properties against enzymatic markers linked with hypertension and diabetes [14].

In another recent study, Karimi et al. [15] investigated the effects of using selective hydrolyzed protein of amaranth on sourdough fermentation, bread quality, and shelf life. Amaranth protein isolate was obtained from defatted amaranth flour using the alkaline extraction-isoelectric precipitation method. Protein hydrolysates were prepared with Alcalase® treatment for 3 h. The authors reported that amaranth protein hydrolysates increased the growth of *Lactobacillus plantarum* and *Saccharomyces cerevisiae* significantly in sourdough compared to amaranth protein isolate and amaranth flour. The use of amaranth protein hydrolysates in the sourdough formulation was indicated to result in changes in dough pH and total titratable acidity after fermentation, as well as changes in specific volume, water activity, and textural characteristics of bread. Sensory properties and shelf life of bread were reported to be improved by the addition of amaranth protein hydrolysates to sourdough [15].

Kiwicha (*Amaranthus caudatus*) is a less known pseudocereal that is indicated as a good source of protein (~13–19%) with a balanced amino acid profile [16]. The physicochemical and functional properties of kiwicha proteins still remain to be explored. There are only few recent reports in the literature on the biological activities of peptides obtained from kiwicha proteins with enzymatic hydrolysis [17–19].

4. Chia protein

The protein content of chia (*Salvia hispanica* L.) seeds changes between ~19 and 23%, and the major protein fractions are reported as globulins, albumins, glutelins, and prolamins [20]. Segura-Campos [21] characterized chia seed proteins. Protein fractions of albumins, globulins, prolamins, and glutelins were obtained based on the Osborne-type fractionation method. The main protein fraction in chia was reported to be glutelin that showed the highest water absorption and holding capacities. Significant differences were observed in emulsifying and foaming properties of fractions obtained from chia protein [21].

Julio et al. [22] prepared different protein fractions of albumins, globulins, glutelins, and prolamins from chia protein-rich fraction of chia seeds, a by-product of chia oil extraction process. The solubility profile of chia protein-rich fraction, globulins, and prolamins was observed to be similar and made a peak at pH 9.0. On the other hand, maximum solubility was observed at pH 5.0 for glutelin and albumin fractions. Detailed emulsion characterization tests including destabilization kinetics and particle size distributions revealed that globulin fraction resulted in the most stable emulsion systems. The authors reported that higher pH values resulted in improved stability in emulsions stabilized with globulins, glutelins, and chia protein-rich fraction [22].

Urbizo-Reyes et al. [23] prepared chia protein hydrolysates with ultrasound treatment followed by microwave-assisted hydrolysis. For this purpose, chia seed mucilage and chia seed oil were extracted from the seeds prior to protein hydrolysis. Chia protein hydrolysates were prepared using Alcalase® or sequential hydrolysis with Alcalase® and Flavourzyme®. Enzymatic hydrolysis reaction was conducted using a conventional or microwave-assisted system. Chia protein hydrolysates obtained using sequential hydrolysis with microwave treatment were reported to show significantly higher *in vitro* antioxidant activity. Hydrolysates were also indicated to show antidiabetic and antihypertensive activities. Microwave treatment during hydrolysis was reported to improve the solubility profile, emulsifying and foaming properties of hydrolysates [23].

5. Teff protein

Teff (*Eragrostis tef*) contains ~13–21% protein with major fractions of glutelin, albumin, and prolamins [24]. Compared to commonly studied proteins from pseudocereal grains, including quinoa, amaranth, and chia, teff proteins remain to be explored in terms of functionality. Gebru et al. [24] studied the variations in amino acid profile and protein composition of white and brown teff seeds during protein extraction. Three different methods were used to obtain fractions of albumins, globulins, prolamins, and glutelins from teff seed flour. White and brown teff seeds were indicated to undergo different changes during protein extraction. Moreover, the essential amino acid content of brown teff seeds was reported to be significantly higher than that of white seeds. Extraction with tert-butanol was indicated to increase prolamin yield compared to extraction with ethanol. Glutelin was reported to be the major protein fraction in both seeds, with white seeds containing higher amounts of glutelin compared to brown seeds. The electrophoretic profile of storage proteins was observed to be different indicating the genetic variations between white and brown teff seeds [24].

Teff flour is widely used in formulations of gluten-free bread and bakery products. Adebowale et al. [25] compared the characteristics of protein fractions in three different teff types with sorghum with the main focus on bread-making quality. The major protein fraction in teff was reported to be prolamin. Aqueous alcohol-soluble protein fraction was indicated to be rich in glutamine and leucine. The authors suggested that differences in the electrophoretic profile of proteins indicated that teff prolamin is less polymerized compared to sorghum prolamin. Functional properties of teff prolamins useful in bread making were attributed to the differences in thermal profile, lower polymerization, and hydrophobicity [25].

6. Buckwheat protein

Common buckwheat (*Fagopyrum esculentum*) and tartary buckwheat (*Fagopyrum tataricum*) are indicated as good sources of protein (8–18% protein) with a balanced amino acid profile [3, 26]. The major storage protein in buckwheat seeds is reported to be 13S globulin [27] and the main protein fractions were reported as albumin, globulin, and glutelin [3]. Functional and bioactive properties of buckwheat protein were recently reviewed by Jin et al. [3]. Tomotake et al. [28] compared the physicochemical and functional properties of buckwheat protein with soy protein isolate and casein. Buckwheat protein was obtained from buckwheat flour using the alkaline extraction-isoelectric precipitation method. Solubility of buckwheat protein was significantly higher than that of soy protein at pH 2.0–10.0, but lower compared to casein at pH 7.0–10.0. The stability of emulsions stabilized by buckwheat protein was observed to be lower compared to soy protein and casein-stabilized emulsions at pH 7.0–10.0. Moreover, the water holding capacity of buckwheat protein was found to be lower than that of soy protein [28].

Xue et al. [29] investigated the effects of high-intensity ultrasound treatment and Maillard reaction on structural, interfacial, and emulsifying properties of buckwheat protein. Buckwheat protein isolate was prepared from defatted buckwheat flour with alkaline extraction method followed by isoelectric precipitation. Buckwheat protein isolate-dextran conjugates were prepared via Maillard reaction combined with ultrasound treatment. The secondary and tertiary structures and surface hydrophobicity of buckwheat protein isolate-dextran conjugates obtained with ultrasonication were observed to be different than those of conjugates obtained with classical heating. As a result of the modifications in protein structure, emulsifying properties and surface activity of conjugates obtained with ultrasonication were reported to be improved compared to classical heating [29].

In another recent study, Wu et al. [30] investigated the effect of extraction pH on structure, functional properties, and digestibility of tartary buckwheat protein. Protein isolates were prepared from defatted tartary buckwheat flour using alkaline extraction at different pH values (pH 7.0–13.0) followed by isoelectric precipitation. Tartary buckwheat flour and protein isolates were separated into albumin, globulin, prolamin, and glutenin fractions based on Osborne-type protein fractionation. Protein extraction at alkaline conditions was reported to increase protein extraction yield. Increased extraction pH was indicated to decrease the albumin content of tartary buckwheat protein isolate while glutenin content increased. The solubility of isolates extracted at pH > 12.0 was observed to decrease. On the other hand, emulsion stability increased at the same conditions that were attributed to increased surface hydrophobicity. The differences observed in *in vitro* digestibility of tartary buckwheat protein isolates obtained at different pH values were related to the modifications in protein structure. The highest digestive rate was observed in isolates obtained at pH 7.0 and 8.0 [30].

In addition to functional properties, buckwheat protein and derived bioactive peptides are reported to show various biological properties, including cholesterol-lowering activity, blood pressure controlling enzyme inhibitory activity, antimicrobial and antioxidant activities that suggest the potential use of buckwheat protein and peptides as functional food ingredients [3].

7. Cañihua protein

Cañihua (*Chenopodium pallidicaule* Aellen), is a less known pseudocereal, contains ~14–19% protein and a balanced essential amino acid profile that are comparable to other commonly known pseudocereals, such as quinoa and amaranth [31].

The major protein fractions in cañihua are reported as albumin and globulin [32]. Betalleluz-Pallardel et al. [33] used response surface methodology for optimization of protein extraction conditions from defatted cañihua grain meal aiming maximized protein extraction yield. Simultaneous effects of pH (7.0–11.0), temperature (25–60°C), solvent:meal ratio (10:1–40:1), time (10–60 min), and NaCl concentration (0–2 M) on protein extraction yield were investigated. Optimum protein extraction conditions were determined as pH 10.0, 21°C, 37:1 (v/w) solvent:meal ratio, and 5 min of extraction time, which resulted in ~80% protein extraction yield [33].

Enzymatic hydrolysis was applied to cañihua protein for obtaining peptides with biological activities. Chirinos et al. [34] derived hydrolysates and peptides from cañihua protein concentrate. Protein concentrate (79% protein) was obtained from defatted cañihua meal with alkaline extraction-isoelectric precipitation method. Cañihua protein concentrate was subjected to enzymatic hydrolysis with Alcalase®, Neutrase®, and Flavourzyme® at 50°C up to 240 min. The hydrolysates obtained were purified via ultrafiltration and size exclusion chromatography to obtain three peptide fractions. The authors reported that cañihua protein can be considered as a good source of bioactive peptides with antioxidant and angiotensin-I converting enzyme (ACE) inhibitory activities. Specifically, cañihua protein hydrolysate obtained with Neutrase®-Alcalase® sequential hydrolysis for 180 min was indicated to show good *in vitro* bioactivity. Two of the purified peptide fractions composed of 3–11 amino acids were indicated to show good *in vitro* antioxidant and antihypertensive activity [34].

In another recent study, Moscoso-Mujica et al. [35] also applied enzymatic hydrolysis to cañihua protein. Cañihua flour was obtained from the seeds of two different varieties (Ramis and Cupi-Sayhua) and defatted prior to protein extraction. Protein fractions of albumins, 7S globulins, 11S globulins, and glutelins were obtained based on solubility differences and subjected to sequential hydrolysis with Alcalase® and pepsin-pancreatin. Hydrolysates with varying degrees of hydrolysis were obtained and tested for antimicrobial activity against *Escherichia coli*, *Staphylococcus aureus*, and *Candida albicans*. The authors reported that among the 216 hydrolysates obtained, only 28 showed significant antimicrobial activity. It was suggested that antimicrobial peptides obtained from fractions of globulins and glutelins can potentially be utilized as novel nutraceutical ingredients [35].

8. Conclusion

Pseudocereals are indicated as good protein sources with a balanced amino acid profile. Nutritional composition and protein characteristics of pseudocereal grains change depending on the seed variety and growing conditions. Moreover, the methods used for protein extraction and fractionation affect protein structure, composition, and hence, functionality. Enzymatic hydrolysis has been shown to be a useful tool for obtaining peptides from pseudocereal proteins with biological activities, including antioxidant, antimicrobial, and antihypertensive properties. Proteins and peptides from pseudocereal grains can be potentially utilized as ingredients in innovative product formulations due to their nutritional quality, functional properties, and biological activities. More research is needed to investigate the effects of pseudocereal proteins on end-product quality to elucidate the potential and increase the utilization of pseudocereal proteins as food ingredients.

Conflict of interest

The author declares no conflicts of interest.

Author details

Asli Can Karaca
Faculty of Chemical and Metallurgical Engineering, Department of Food Engineering, Istanbul Technical University, Istanbul, Turkey

*Address all correspondence to: cankaraca@itu.edu.tr

References

[1] López DN, Galante M, Robson M, Boeris V, Spelzini D. Amaranth, quinoa and chia protein isolates: Physicochemical and structural properties. International Journal of Biological Macromolecules. 2018;**109**:152-159. DOI: 10.1016/j.ijbiomac.2017.12.080

[2] Dakhili S, Abdolalizadeh L, Hosseini SM, Shojaee-Aliabadi S, Mirmoghtadaie L. Quinoa protein: Composition, structure and functional properties. Food Chemistry. 2019;**299**:125161. DOI: 10.1016/j.foodchem.2019.125161

[3] Jin J, Ohanenye IC, Udenigwe CC. Buckwheat proteins: Functionality, safety, bioactivity, and prospects as alternative plant-based proteins in the food industry. Critical Reviews in Food Science and Nutrition. 2020. DOI: 10.1080/10408398.2020.1847027

[4] Schmidt D, Verruma-Bernardi MR, Forti VA, Borges MTMR. Quinoa and amaranth as functional foods: A review. Food Reviews International. 2021:1-20. DOI: 10.1080/87559129.2021.1950175

[5] Abugoch LE, Romero N, Tapia CA, Silva J, Rivera M. Study of some physicochemical and functional properties of quinoa (*Chenopodium Quinoa* Willd) protein isolates. Journal of Agricultural and Food Chemistry. 2008;**56**:4745-4750. DOI: 10.1021/jf703689u

[6] Van de Vondel J, Lambrecht MA, Delcour JA. Heat-induced denaturation and aggregation of protein in quinoa (*Chenopodium quinoa* Willd.) seeds and whole meal. Food Chemistry. 2022;**372**:131330. DOI: 10.1016/j.foodchem.2021.131330

[7] Guo H, Hao Y, Yang X, Ren G, Richel A. Exploration on bioactive properties of quinoa protein hydrolysate and peptides: A review. Critical Reviews in Food Science and Nutrition. 2021. DOI: 10.1080/10408398.2021.1982860

[8] Daliri H, Ahmadi R, Pezeshki A, Hamishehkar H, Mohammadi M, Beyrami H, et al. Quinoa bioactive protein hydrolysate produced by pancreatin enzyme- functional and antioxidant properties. LWT. 2021;**150**:111853. DOI: 10.1016/j.lwt.2021.111853

[9] Teng C, Xing B, Fan X, Zhang B, Li Y, Ren G. Effects of Maillard reaction on the properties and anti-inflammatory, anti-proliferative activity in vitro of quinoa protein isolates. Industrial Crops and Products. 2021;**174**:114165. DOI: 10.1016/j.indcrop.2021.114165

[10] Condés MC, Scilingo AA, Añón MC. Characterization of amaranth proteins modified by trypsin proteolysis. Structural and functional changes. LWT-Food Science and Technology. 2009;**42**:963-970. DOI: 10.1016/j.lwt.2008.12.008

[11] Tömösközi S, Gyenge L, Pelceder A, Varga J, Abonyi T, Lasztity R. Functional properties of protein preparations from amaranth seeds in model system. European Food Research and Technology. 2008;**226**:1343-1348. DOI: 10.1007/s00217-007-0663-3

[12] Figueroa-González JJ, Lobato-Calleros C, Vernon-Carter EJ, Aguirre-Mandujano E, Alvarez-Ramirez J, Martínez-Velasco A. Modifying the structure, physicochemical properties, and foaming ability of amaranth protein by dual pH-shifting and ultrasound

treatments. LWT. 2022;**153**:112561. DOI: 10.1016/j.lwt.2021.112561

[13] Das D, Mir NA, Chandla NK, Singh S. Combined effect of pH treatment and the extraction pH on the physicochemical, functional and rheological characteristics of amaranth (*Amaranthus hypochondriacus*) seed protein isolates. Food Chemistry. 2021;**353**:129466. DOI: 10.1016/j.foodchem.2021.129466

[14] Kamal H, Mudgil P, Bhaskar B, Fisayo AF, Gan CY, Maqsood S. Amaranth proteins as potential source of bioactive peptides with enhanced inhibition of enzymatic markers linked with hypertension and diabetes. Journal of Cereal Science. 2021;**101**:103308. DOI: 10.1016/j.jcs.2021.103308

[15] Karimi N, Zeynali F, Bari MR, Nikoo M, Mohtarami F, Kadivar M. Amaranth selective hydrolyzed protein influence on sourdough fermentation and wheat bread quality. Food Science & Nutrition. 2021;**9**:6683-6691. DOI: 10.1002/fsn3.2618

[16] Martinez-Lopez A, Millan-Linares MC, Rodriguez-Martin NM, Millan F, Montserrat-de la Paz S. Nutraceutical value of kiwicha (*Amaranthus caudatus* L.). Journal of Functional Foods. 2020;**65**:103735. DOI: 10.1016/j.jff.2019.103735

[17] Vilcacundo R, Martinez-Villaluenga C, Miralles B, Hernandez-Ledesma B. Release of multifunctional peptides from kiwicha (*Amaranthus caudatus*) protein under in vitro gastrointestinal digestion. Journal of the Science of Food and Agriculture. 2019;**99**:1225-1232. DOI: 10.1002/jsfa.9294

[18] Chirinos R, Pedreschi R, Velasquez-Sanchez M, Aguilar-Galvez A, Campos D. In vitro antioxidant and angiotensin I-converting enzyme inhibitory properties of enzymatically hydrolyzed quinoa (*Chenopodium quinoa*) and kiwicha (*Amaranthus caudatus*) proteins. Cereal Chemistry. 2020;**97**:949-957. DOI: 10.1002/cche.10317

[19] Montserrat-de la Paz S, Martinez-Lopez A, Villanueva-Lazo A, Pedroche J, Millan F, Millan-Linares MC. Identification and characterization of novel antioxidant protein hydrolysates from kiwicha (*Amaranthus caudatus* L.). Antioxidants. 2021;**10**:645. DOI: 10.3390/antiox10050645

[20] Salazar-Vega IM, Julio LM, Segura-Campos MR, Tomas MC. Chia protein hydrolysates: Characterisation and emulsifying properties. International Journal of Food Science and Technology. 2021;**56**:3546-3555. DOI: 10.1111/ijfs.14981

[21] Segura-Campos MR. Isolation and functional caharacterization of chia (*Salvia hispanica*) proteins. Food Science and Technology. 2020;**40**:334-339. DOI: 10.1590/fst.41618

[22] Julio LM, Ruiz-Ruiz JC, Tomas MC, Segura-Campos MR. Chia (*Salvia hispanica*) protein fractions: Characterization and emulsifying properties. Journal of Food Measurement and Characterization. 2019;**13**:3318-3328. DOI: 10.1007/s11694-019-00254-w

[23] Urbizo-Reyes U, San Martin-González MF, Garcia-Bravo J, Malo Vigil AL, Liceaga AM. Physicochemical characteristics of chia seed (*Salvia hispanica*) protein hydrolysates produced using ultrasonication followed by microwave-assisted hydrolysis. Food Hydrocolloids. 2019;**97**:105187. DOI: 10.1016/j.foodhyd.2019.105187

[24] Gebru YA, Jun H, Young-Soo K, Myung-Kon K, Kwang-Pyo K. Variations in amino acid and protein profiles in

white versus brown teff (*Eragrostis Tef*) seeds, and effect of extraction methods on protein yields. Food. 2019;**8**:202. DOI: 10.3390/foods8060202

[25] Adebowale ARA, Emmambux MN, Beukes M, Taylor JRN. Fractionation and characterization of teff proteins. Journal of Cereal Science. 2011;**54**:380-386. DOI: 10.1016/j.jcs.2011.08.002

[26] Luthar Z, Zhou M, Golob A, Germ M. Breeding buckwheat for increased levels and improved quality of protein. Plants. 2021;**10**:14. DOI: 10.3390/plants10010014

[27] Radovic SR, Maksimovic VR, Varkonji-Gasic EI. Characterization of buckwheat seed storage proteins. Journal of Agricultural and Food Chemistry. 1996;**44**:972-974. DOI: 10.1021/jf950655x

[28] Tomotake H, Shimaoka I, Kayashita J, Nakajoh M, Kato N. Physicochemical and functional properties of buckwheat protein product. Journal of Agricultural and Food Chemistry. 2002;**50**:2125-2129. DOI: 10.1021/jf011248q

[29] Xue F, Wu Z, Tong J, Zheng J, Li C. Effect of combination of high-intensity ultrasound treatment and dextran glycosylation on structural and interfacial properties of buckwheat protein isolates. Bioscience, Biotechnology, and Biochemistry. 2017;**81**:1891-1898. DOI: 10.1080/09168451.2017.1361805

[30] Wu L, Li J, Wu W, Wang L, Qin F, Xie W. Effect of extraction pH on functional properties, structural properties, and in vitro gastrointestinal digestion of tartary buckwheat protein isolates. Journal of Cereal Science. 2021;**101**:103314. DOI: 10.1016/j.jcs.2021.103314

[31] Gomez Cahuata JF, Rosas-Quina YE, Pachari Vera E. Cañihua (*Chenopodium pallidicaule* Aellen) a promising superfood in food industry: A review. Nutrition & Food Science. 2021. DOI: 10.1108/NFS-09-2021-0277

[32] Repo-Carrasco R, Espinoza C, Jacobsen S-E. Nutritional value and use of the Andean crops quinoa (*Chenopodium quinoa*) and kañiwa (*Chenopodium pallidicaule*). Food Reviews International. 2003;**19**:179-189. DOI: 10.1081/FRI-120018884

[33] Betalleluz-Pallardel I, Inga M, Mera L, Pedreschi R, Campos D, Chirinos R. Optimisation of extraction conditions and thermal properties ofprotein from the Andean pseudocereal cañihua (*Chenopodium pallidicaule* Aellen). International Journal of Food Science and Technology. 2017;**52**:1026-1034. DOI: 10.1111/ijfs.13368

[34] Chirinos R, Ochoa K, Aguilar-Galvez A, Carpentier S, Pedreschi R, Campos D. Obtaining of peptides with in vitro antioxidant and angiotensin I converting enzyme inhibitory activities from cañihua protein (*Chenopodium pallidicaule* Aellen). Journal of Cereal Science. 2018;**83**:139-146. DOI: 10.1016/j.jcs.2018.07.004

[35] Moscoso-Mujica G, Zavaleta AI, Mujica A, Arnao I, Moscoso-Neira C, Santos M, et al. Antimicrobial peptides purified from hydrolysates of kanihua (*Chenopodium pallidicaule* Aellen) seed protein fractions. Food Chemistry. 2021;**360**:129951. DOI: 10.1016/j.foodchem.2021.129951

Chapter 4

Pseudocereals: A Novel Path towards Healthy Eating

Upasana and Latika Yadav

Abstract

Nowadays, interest in research about pseudocereals has increased worldwide. Pseudocereals can be defined as seeds or fruits of non-grass species that can be consumed similarly to cereals. The most extensively used pseudocereals include quinoa, chia, buckwheat, amaranth, and so on. All of them, have good nutritional and bioactive compounds such as essential amino acids, essential fatty acids, phenolic acids, flavonoids, minerals, and vitamins. Food and Agriculture Organization (FAO) has also reported that there is a buddle of plants that are under-utilized that significantly contribute to improving nutrition and health as well as enhancing food basket and livelihoods of the individual; contributing to future food security and sustainability. Earlier studies also reported that pseudocereals protein-derived peptides have anti-cancerous, anti-inflammatory, anti-hypertensive, hypocholesterolemic, and antioxidant properties. The presence of these interesting properties in pseudocereals enhances the interest to carry out extensive research regarding their health benefits and the way to incorporate them into the diet. In this chapter, we portray different types of pseudocereals with their nutritional benefits for living a healthy and active life.

Keywords: amaranth, buckwheat, chia, quinoa, pseudocereals

1. Introduction

Food grains play a pivotal role in maintaining a healthy and active lifestyle. Every food has distinctiveness in its composition with a wide variety of macro and micronutrients in a different composition. Food grains that are rich sources of carbohydrates (rice, wheat, maize, etc.), protein (pulses, legumes, etc.), fats (groundnut, oilseeds), or minerals (pearl millet, etc.), while some are nutrient-dense and have optimum combinations of nutrients with good digestibility (most of the minor millets, quinoa, etc.) [1]. These nutrient-dense food grains are an adequate mix of nutrients with good bioavailability. On the other hand, pseudocereals are considered as "sub-exploited foods" or "under-utilized foods" defined as food groups that comprise non-grasses plant species not belonging to the cereals family but with similar properties and uses [1].

Currently, interest is arising regarding the use of an alternative source of cereals that can be pertinent to multiple reasons. All over the world, there is a bang regarding gathering knowledge about healthy eating options and incorporating it into the diet. Several trending terms are floating on the internet, magazines, books like healthy, wholesome, natural, or minimally processed and within cereals; for example, wholegrain, gluten-free, rich in dietary fiber or resistant starch, low carb, or digestibility have arisen and so on [2]. In the above context, pseudocereals fit properly as well as acknowledged for their several health benefits. Elevated consumption of pseudocereals for human consumption leads the food producers to develop novel and convenient food products which require not only know-how about the chemical composition of these raw materials, but also fundamental information about their physical and functional properties for processing [2].

Since agriculture is considered a cornerstone of the nation and therefore utilizing a handful of crops has placed global food security at risk [3]. Presently, the agro-industry is facing a crisis to assure adequate food supply to the 7 billion population of the world by maintaining high productivity and quality standards [3]. To confront this problem, a multidisciplinary approach is required to strengthen the food basket as well as make access to nutritious foods through nutritional supplements, enrichment, biofortification, and so on which act as a backbone of food security. The mentioned facts infuriate the researchers and scientists to explore and disseminate the knowledge regarding sub-exploited foods. These grains are rich in high-quality proteins, starch, minerals, vitamins, bioactive compounds, and nutraceuticals. This composition elaborates the potential of pseudocereals to replace or supplement conventionally utilized cereals. Since the content of gluten is also either very low or

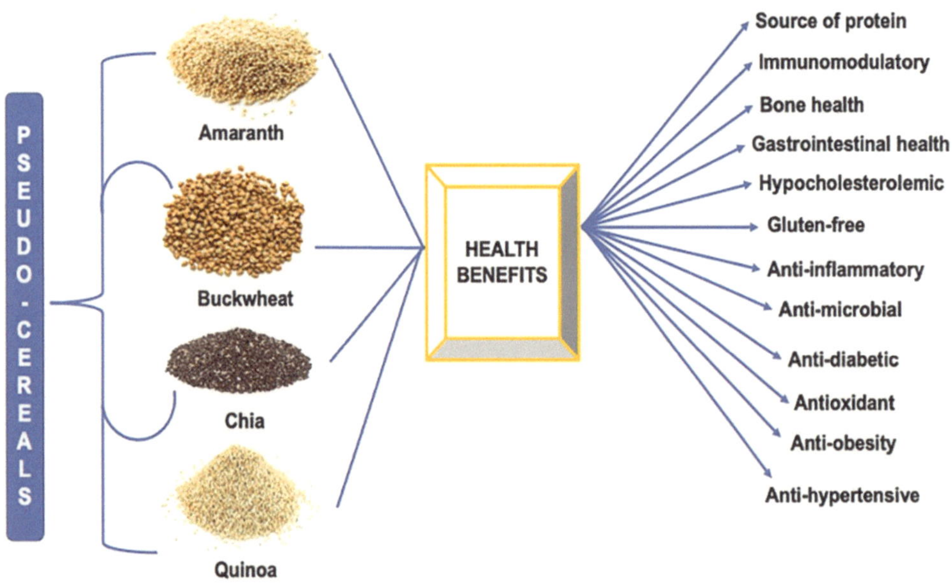

Figure 1.
Health benefits of pseudocereals. The figure was modified from the following research paper by Thakur et al. [5]. The images used in drawing the figure were extracted from the following links as described below: 1. Amaranth: https://rukminim1.flixcart.com/image/416/416/kh9gbrk0/edible-seed/7/z/n/900-pouch-raw-farmory-whole-original-imafxbhkzpnxkwky.jpeg?q=70, 2. Buckwheat: https://m.media-amazon.com/images/I/71XHdM6NAvL._SL1000_.jpg, 3. Chia: https://img1.exportersindia.com/product_images/bc-full/dir_79/2366770/organic-chia-seeds-2398993.jpeg, 4. Quinoa: https://4.imimg.com/data4/BL/DW/MY-24035409/white-quinoa-seed-500x500.jpg.

gluten-free; it can be incorporated in celiac diseases as well as also various health benefits [4]. This chapter is designed to portray the different variety of pseudocereals with their health benefits that ultimately pave the path towards healthy living which is well depicted in **Figure 1**.

2. Types of pseudocereals

In the human diet, pseudocereals play a remarkable role to meet the necessities of the population suffering from coeliac diseases as well as other health consequences due to their wide range of nutrients like carbohydrates, proteins, fats, vitamins, minerals, and nutraceuticals. Here, in this chapter mainly four types of pseudocereals are discussed namely amaranth, buckwheat, chia seeds, and quinoa. These pseudocereals are discussed below:

2.1 Amaranth

Amaranth is known as one of the New World's oldest crops, originated in Mesoamerica [6]. It is a dicotyledonous pseudocereal that belongs to the family of Amaranthaceae. The word Amaranthus is derived from the Greek word "anthos" (flower) which means everlasting or unwilting. Presently, it is widely cultivated and consumed throughout India, Nepal, Southern, and Eastern Africa, Malaysia, Indonesia, Philippines, Central America, and Mexico [6]. The common species of Amaranthus grown for alleviating the dietary beneficiaries for human consumption includes *Amaranthus hypochondriacus, Amaranthus caudatus, Amaranthus cruentus*, and so on.

It is considered a superfood because of its high nutraceutical properties like the high quality of proteins with multiple essential amino acids, a good source of unsaturated fats like omega-3 and omega-6 fatty acids, squalene, tocopherols, phenolic compounds, flavonoids, phytates, vitamins, minerals, and dietary fibers [7] which is well represented from **Tables 1–3**.

Parameters	Amaranth	Buckwheat	Chia	Quinoa
Water (g)	11.3	—	5.8	13.3
Ash (g)	2.88	—	4.8	2.38
Energy (kcal)	371	333	486	368
Protein (g)	13.6	13.3	16.5	14.1
Carbohydrate by difference (g)	65.2	62.2	42.1	64.2
Total lipid/fat (g)	7.02	2.22	30.7	6.07
Fiber, total dietary (g)	6.7	2.2	34.4	7
Fatty acids, total saturated (g)	1.46	0	3.33	0.706
Fatty acids, total monounsaturated (g)	1.68	—	2.31	1.61
Fatty acids, total polyunsaturated (g)	2.78	—	23.7	3.29

Table 1.
Macronutrient's content of amaranth, buckwheat, chia seeds, and quinoa [8–11].

Parameters	Amaranth	Buckwheat	Chia	Quinoa
Calcium, Ca (mg)	159	67	631	47
Iron, Fe (mg)	7.61	2	7.72	4.57
Magnesium, Mg (mg)	248	—	335	197
Phosphorus, P (mg)	557	—	860	457
Potassium, K (mg)	508	311	407	563
Sodium, Na (mg)	4	0	16	5
Zinc, Zn (mg)	2.87	—	4.58	3.1
Copper, Cu (mg)	0.525	—	0.924	0.59
Manganese, Mn (mg)	3.33	—	2.72	2.03
Selenium, Se (μg)	18.7	—	55.2	8.5

Table 2.
Mineral's content of amaranth, buckwheat, chia seeds, and quinoa [8–11].

Parameters	Amaranth	Buckwheat	Chia	Quinoa
Vitamin A (IU)	0	—	54	14
Vitamin B1, Thiamine (mg)	0.116	—	0.62	0.36
Vitamin B2, Riboflavin (mg)	0.2	—	0.17	0.318
Vitamin B3, Niacin (mg)	0.923	—	8.83	1.52
Vitamin B5, Pantothenic acid (mg)	1.46	—	—	0.772
Vitamin B6, Pyridoxine (mg)	0.591	—	—	0.487
Folate, total (μg)	82	—	49	184
Vitamin B12 (μg)	0	—	0	0
Vitamin C (mg)	4.2	—	1.6	—
Vitamin D (IU)	0	0	—	0
Vitamin E (mg)	1.19	—	0.5	2.44
Vitamin K (μg)	0	—	—	1.1

Table 3.
Vitamin's content of amaranth, buckwheat, chia seeds, and quinoa [8–11].

2.1.1 Health benefits of Amaranth

2.1.1.1 Rich source of protein

The grains of amaranth have higher sources of protein especially have a higher content of lysine and tryptophan which is limiting in the conventional cereals like wheat, rice, and maize whereas, it is deficient in leucine. Earlier studies are also stated that the protein content of the amaranth is also relatively rich in sulfur-containing amino acids, which are generally limited in the pulses [12]. Since, it is well known that protein is required for every cell for growth and maintenance of the body, for supporting neurological functions, aids in digestion balances hormones naturally as well as maintaining the immune system [6].

2.1.1.2 Reduces inflammation

It is well known that inflammation is a normal process of immune response designed to protect the body against infection and injury. If the inflammation process exists in the body; this may be contributed to or be associated with diabetes, cancer, or any other autoimmune diseases [6]. It was also elaborated in earlier studies that consumption of amaranth reduces the inflammation caused by diseases. This is so because extruded amaranth protein hydrolysates prevent inflammation by the activation of bioactive peptides that reduces the expression of several pro-inflammatory markers [6, 13].

2.1.1.3 Health of the bone

Calcium is the main driver in maintaining healthy bones in the human body. As the composition suggests, amaranth contains more calcium than any other seeds making them helpful for preventing osteoporosis and many other diseases related to bone health. Therefore, it was stated earlier in the studies that the intake of extruded amaranth products helps individuals in improving and maintaining the optimum calcium requirement for healthy bone density [6].

2.1.1.4 Cholesterol-lowering effect

Previous studies reported that amaranth's oil helps the individual in reducing total and LDL (low-density lipoprotein) cholesterol) as well as increases the HDL (high-density lipoprotein) cholesterol in a tested animal model [6, 14]. Also, it was reported that amaranth affects the absorption of cholesterol and bile acid production, hepatic cholesterol content, distribution of cholesterol lipoprotein, and biosynthesis cholesterol [6, 15].

2.1.1.5 Fights against duodenal peptic ulcers

It was revealed from the earlier studies that the duodenal peptic ulcer and chronic gastritis caused by Helicobacter pylori can be cured with Amaranth oil [7, 16].

2.1.1.6 Fights against diabetes

The incorporation of amaranth helps diabetic patients in regulating the blood glucose level due to its higher content of manganese that helps in the pathway of gluconeogenesis. Besides the above, manganese also helps in maintaining the immune system of the individual, level of cholesterol, skin and bone health as well as the renal function of the individual [7].

2.1.1.7 Gluten-free

Amaranth can be considered as an excellent source of gluten-free protein required for patients of coeliac disease as well as for those who want to incorporate a gluten-free diet into their lifestyle.

2.1.1.8 Helps pregnant women

Since folic acid is suggested to pregnant women to be incorporated in their diet to prevent the birth defects like spina bifida and heart diseases. As the content of amaranth suggests the folic content is 88.0 mcg which is beneficial for the generation of new cells; therefore, helps pregnant women in decreasing the incidence of organism defects [7].

2.1.1.9 Prevents constipation

It is well reported that amaranth is a good source of soluble dietary fibers. As we know dietary fibers aid bowel movements helping the individual in preventing constipation.

2.1.1.10 Antioxidant property

Antioxidants are known as "scavengers of free radicals". These components help in inhibiting oxidation lower the risk of infections, maintain heart health, and prevent several forms of cancers and degenerative diseases. In amaranth, the antioxidant potential is attributed to the presence of phenolics and flavonoids. It was reported that Amaranthus flowers, leaves as well as extracts possess the highest antioxidant activities compared to other parts, rutin being the major radical scavenger [6, 17].

2.1.1.11 Amaranth is a superfood that provides optimum nutrition for maintaining good health

As reported earlier in several studies amaranth supports several physiological processes in the human body by playing the role of antimicrobial, hepato-protective, anti-cancerous, anti-malarial, anti-anemic, supplementary, or nutraceutical foods, and so on. Due to its presence of high content of iron, manganese, calcium, dietary fibers, essential amino acids, lipids, antioxidants, it is labeled as a superfood that is required for sustaining a healthy lifestyle.

2.2 Buckwheat

Buckwheat is also known as gluten-free pseudocereals belongs to the family of Polygonaceae with the genus Fagopyrum. Common buckwheat that is cultivated for human consumption includes *Fagopyrum esculentum* and *Fagopyrum tartaricum*. The significant producer of buckwheat all over the world include Russia, China, and Ukraine. Now a days, its consumption is increasing all over the world. In India, on Hindu traditions during the period of fasting (like Navaratri, Ekadashi, Mahashivaratri, Janmashtami, etc.) people of northern states eat foods made up of buckwheat flour; as eating cereals made up of wheat, rice, maize is prohibited during fasting days [18].

Buckwheat is considered as a good source of nutrients like proteins, fats, vitamins (like B1, B2, B3, and B6), minerals (like copper, zinc, manganese, selenium, sodium, potassium, calcium, magnesium), dietary fibers, and in combination with other health-promoting components like organic acids, polyphenols, flavonoids and inositol [19]. Due to its composition of the high biological value of proteins and amino acids, it is considered superior to other grains which are well shown in **Tables 1–3**.

2.2.1 Health benefits of buckwheat

2.2.1.1 Antioxidant effects

Buckwheat contains antioxidants including flavonoids like oligomeric proanthocyanidins which are found in hulls and seeds as well as present in buckwheat flour.

It also contains protective phenolic compounds that help in fighting against cancer or heart diseases [20]. Moreover, antioxidants also support cellular functions of the body by protecting DNA from damage and preventing inflammation or cancerous cell formation [20].

2.2.1.2 Source of highly digestible protein

It is well known that proteins are known as "building blocks" as it is required for the growth, development, and maintenance of the body. As stated earlier in the studies buckwheat is a good source of protein as it contains almost 12 amino acids as compared to conventional cereals like rice, wheat, or maize. Furthermore, buckwheat also contains essential amino acids like lysine and arginine that ensure the full range of amino acids required for the proper functioning of the human body [20]. The grains of buckwheat contain roughly 11–14 grams of protein for every 100 grams which are almost higher than most whole grains [20].

2.2.1.3 Source of dietary fibers

It was reported previously that 1 cup serving of buckwheat provides almost 6 gm of dietary fibers; which helps to fill you up and hastens the transit of food through the digestive tract (essential for bowel movement regulation). Moreover, buckwheat also protects the digestive organs from infections, cancers as well as other negative symptoms by preventing oxidative stress within the gastrointestinal tract [20].

2.2.1.4 Anti-diabetic effects

Buckwheat has a low glycemic index as compared to other conventional cereals like rice, wheat, and maize. It possesses anti-nutritional factors like polyphenols and enzyme-inhibitors that delay digestion; thus, helping in regulating the blood glucose level [19]. Previously, it was also stated that buckwheat contains rutin and quercetin that helps in reducing insulin resistance conditions by enhancing the capability of hepatic antioxidant enzymes [19, 21]. Nevertheless, it was also revealed from the study that the chemically synthesized D-chiro-inositol (an insulin regulatory component) is used to lower serum glucose concentrations in diabetic patients and is available relatively in high amounts in buckwheat [19, 22].

2.2.1.5 Gluten-free and non-allergic

The size, appearance, texture, and taste of buckwheat are very similar to barley but the main advantage of buckwheat is zero gluten [20]. As a result, buckwheat is safe for individuals suffering from coeliac diseases or for individuals who want to take a gluten-free diet. It also helps in preventing numerous diseases related to the gastrointestinal tract like diarrhea, bloating, constipation, leaky gut syndrome, and so on.

2.2.1.6 Furnishes important minerals and vitamins

The flours of buckwheat contain minerals like iron, zinc, phosphorus, magnesium, manganese, and folate as well as contains vitamins like B vitamins. It was elaborated that the manganese content of buckwheat helps in improving the digestion process, aid in muscle growth and recovery, and defend against stress's negative impacts on the body [20]. Nevertheless, B vitamins, manganese, phosphorus, and zinc help the individual in maintaining healthy circulation and blood vessel function, plus they are needed for neurotransmitter signaling in the brain that fights depression, anxiety, and headaches [20].

2.2.1.7 Other benefits

Several studies reported that buckwheat plays multiple roles in regulating numerous physiological processes by acting as a hypocholesterolemic, hypotensive, hypoglycaemic, neuroprotective, anti-obesity agent as well as anti-aging foods.

2.3 Chia seeds

Chia seeds are originated from Mexico, belong to the family Lamiaceae with the representative of genus Salvia and species hispanica. The chia seeds are utilized in the form of whole seeds, flour, mucilage as well as seed oil. It is a nutrient-dense superfood that contains superior quality omega-3 fatty acids, gluten-free protein, and high content of anti-oxidants protecting seeds against microbial and chemical degradations [23, 24]. It is an oilseed that contains carbohydrates, proteins, lipids, dietary fibers, vitamins, minerals, and phytochemicals which is well shown in **Tables 1–3**.

2.3.1 Health benefits of chia seeds

2.3.1.1 Gluten-free

Likewise, other pseudocereals, chia seed is also gluten-free; so, these can be incorporated by individuals who are suffering from health issues like gluten intolerance.

2.3.1.2 Protein content

It is well known that protein is a macronutrient, utilized by the body for the generation of energy to perform multiple body functions [23]. Chia seeds possess a significant amount of protein that helps in minimizing the problem of protein-energy malnutrition [23, 25]. Previous studies also enumerated that chia seeds possess an excellent balance of amino acids containing a high concentration of cysteine, lysine, and methionine as compared to the primary cereals [23, 26]. Another study reported that regular consumption of chia seeds having an appreciable amount of protein in the diet proved helpful for the individual suffering from either obesity or overweight and other health-related issues such as diabetes [23, 27].

2.3.1.3 Antioxidant

It is well known that antioxidants are the components that have the potential to neutralize the free radical and thus help the individual in preventing various metabolic disorders. From various clinical studies, it was revealed that chia seeds are a potential source of antioxidants like sterols, tocopherols, and polyphenolic compounds like caffeic acid, myricetin, chlorogenic acid, protocatechuic acid, quercetin, kaempferol, rutin, and so on; exhibits beneficial effects like anti-aging, anti-carcinogenic, neuroprotective, cardioprotective, hepatoprotective as well as prevent some neurological disorders.

2.3.1.4 Dietary fibers

Dietary fiber is an important constituent of our diet. According to recommended dietary allowances 2020, it was prescribed to include 25 gm for sedentary women and 32 gm for sedentary men of dietary fiber per day [28]. It was stated in the previous study that the fiber content of chia seeds is almost twice as bran, 4–5 times greater than amaranth, quinoa, soya, and almonds [29]. Several clinical studies stated that optimum intake of dietary fibers helps the individual from several disorders like diseases related to the digestive and circulatory system, hemorrhoids, kidney stones, colorectal cancer, diabetes mellitus, metabolic diseases, and so on.

2.4 Quinoa

Quinoa is an annual herbaceous, dicotyledonous plant belonging to the Chenopodiaceae family with the genus with the genus Chenopodium and species quinoa. It is originated in the Andean region and able to adapt to different climatic conditions and soils [30]. This pseudocereal is a rich source of proteins with an exceptional balance of essential amino acids, fats, vitamins, minerals, and fibers which is well depicted in **Tables 1**–**3**. It also contains health-beneficial phytochemicals like saponins, phytosterols, and phtoecdysteroids [30]. Above all, it contains top-level protein i.e., lysine and methionine when compared to conventional cereals like wheat, rice, maize, barley [31]. It was also reported in previous studies that the fatty acid composition of quinoa is almost equivalent to soyabean oil [31].

2.4.1 Health benefits of quinoa

2.4.1.1 Good for celiac diseases

Celiac disease is a condition in which an individual is not able to tolerate the gluten protein which is found in traditional cereals like wheat, rye, barley, and so on. It is well known that quinoa is free from gluten protein; so, it is well tolerated by patients with celiac diseases as well as for individuals who want to include gluten-free food products in their diet.

2.4.1.2 Antioxidant property

Reported in earlier studies that the main edible part of the quinoa plant is quinoa seeds, but the leaves too contain rich phenolic compounds that have antioxidant and anti-cancerous properties [32]. The quinoa extracts contain a considerable amount of ferulic, sinapinic, and gallic acids, kaempferol, isorhamnetin, and rutin an inhibitory effect on prostate cancer cell proliferation and motility [32, 33]. It has been also proposed that these compounds help in reducing the risk of neurodegenerative disorders, cardiovascular diseases as well as diabetes [32–34].

2.4.1.3 Anti-diabetic, anti-obesity, and hypocholesterolemic effect

Various clinical studies elaborated that quinoa contains multiple types of bioactive components like peptides, polysaccharides, phenolics, phytosterols, and so on that are proposed to prevent health complications like hyperglycemia, adiposity, and dyslipidemia. The mechanism involved for the above beneficial effects includes reduced lipid absorption and adipogenesis, increased energy expenditure and glucose oxidation, and corrected gut microbiota [35]. It can be stated that quinoa offers several unique attributes that could be harnessed to improve the dietary management of obesity, diabetes as well as cardiovascular diseases [35].

3. Conclusion

The innovation of nutraceutical foods and its product is one of the captivating shifts of agri-food industries. With the growing awareness of individuals regarding nutritious foods all over the world; the burden arises for researchers and scientists to develop food products that are high in protein content, gluten-free as well as nutrient-dense. As a result, in the last couple of years, interest arouses regarding the development of nutritious healthy products from pseudocereals for living a disease-free and healthy life; that can be beneficial for coeliac patients as well. As we know amaranth, buckwheat, chia seeds as well as quinoa are the major pseudocereals that have a balanced nutrient composition of dietary protein, fats, vitamins, minerals, dietary fibers, antioxidants as well as bioactive components that have beneficial properties like cardioprotective, immunomodulatory, anti-diabetic, anti-obesity, anti-inflammatory, hypocholesterolemic, maintains disorders of the gastrointestinal tract and so on. The gluten-free products which are available in the market are prepared by using starches and additives that are deficient in vital nutrients which are required for the growth and development of individuals suffering from coeliac disease. Therefore, incorporation of these gluten-free pseudocereals (amaranth, buckwheat, chia seeds, and quinoa) in the diet of coeliac patients not only pacifies the nutrient deficiency but also paves the path of blossoming these underutilized food grains.

Acknowledgements

We pay our profound sense of gratitude to Mr. Nirmal Kumar for his assistance, encouragement, and insightful advice throughout in constructing this book chapter. We also apologize for not citing the research papers of all the authors that helped us in better understanding of this topic.

Conflict of interest

Authors declare no conflict of interest.

Author details

Upasana[1*] and Latika Yadav[2]

1 Mahila College Dalmianagar, Rohtas, Veer Kunwar Singh University, Ara, Bihar, India

2 Government Degree College, Puwarka, Saharanpur, Uttar Pradesh, India

*Address all correspondence to: me.upasana87@gmail.com

References

[1] Rodriguez JP, Rahman H, Thushar S, Singh RK. Healthy and resilient cereals and Pseudo-cereals for marginal agriculture: Molecular advances for improving nutrient bioavailability. Frontiers in Genetics. 27 Feb 2020;**11**: 1-29. DOI: 10.3389/fgene.2020.00049

[2] Bender D, Schonlechner R. Recent developments and knowledge in pseudocereals including technological aspects. Acta Alimentaria. 20 Jul 2021;**50**(4):583-609. DOI: 10.1556/066.2021.00136

[3] Pirzadah TB, Malik B. Pseudocereals as super foods of 21st century: Recent technological interventions. Journal of Agriculture and Food Research. Dec 2020;**2**:100052. DOI: 10.1016/j.jafr.2020.100052

[4] Stamatovska V, Nakov G, Uzunoska Z, Kalevska T, Menkinoska M. Potential use of some pseudocereals in the food industry. ARTTE. Jan 2018;**6**(1):54-61. DOI: 10.15547/artte.2018.01.009

[5] Thakur P, Kumar K, Dhaliwal HS. Nutritional facts, bioactive components and processing aspects of pseudocereals: A comprehensive review. Food Bioscience. 2021;**42**:101170. DOI: 10.1016/j.fbio.2021.101170

[6] Soriano-Garcia M, Aguirre-Diaz IS. Nutritional functional value and therapeutic utilization of Amaranth. In: Waisundara VY, editor. Nutritional Value of Amaranth. London: IntechOpen; 2019. DOI: 10.5772/intechopen.86897. Available from: https://www.intechopen.com/chapters/67741

[7] Soriano-Garcia M, Ilnamiqui I, Arias-Olguin MJPC, Ramírez DGR, Figueroa JSM, Flores-Valverde E, et al. Nutritional functional value and therapeutic utilization of Amaranth. Journal of Analytical & Pharmaceutical Research. 23 Oct 2018;7(5):596-600. DOI: 10.15406/japlr.2018.07.00288

[8] Amaranth grain, uncooked: Food data central, U.S. Department of Agriculture. Available from: https://fdc.nal.usda.gov/fdc-app.html#/food-details/170682/nutrients [Accessed: January 27, 2022]

[9] Raw Buckwheat Groats: Food data central, U.S. Department of Agriculture. Available from: https://fdc.nal.usda.gov/fdc-app.html#/food-details/1013209/nutrients [Accessed: January 27, 2022]

[10] Seeds, Chia seeds, dried: Food data central, U.S. Department of Agriculture. Available from: https://fdc.nal.usda.gov/fdc-app.html#/food-details/170554/nutrients [Accessed: January 27, 2022]

[11] Quinoa, uncooked: Food data central, U.S. Department of Agriculture. Available from: https://fdc.nal.usda.gov/fdc-app.html#/food-details/168874/nutrients [Accessed: January 27, 2022]

[12] Maurya NK, Arya P. Amaranthus grain nutritional benefits: A review. Journal of Pharmacognosy and Phytochemistry. 2018;7(2):2258-2262

[13] Montoya-Rodrguez A, de Mejja EG, Dia VP, Reyes-Moreno C, Milan-Carrillo J. Extrusion improved the anti-inflammatory effect of amaranth (Amaranthus hypochondriacus) hydrolysates in LPS-induced human THP-1 macrophage-like and mouse RAW 264.7 macrophages by preventing activation of NF-κB signaling. Molecular Nutrition & Food Research. May 2014;**58**(5):1028-1041. DOI: 10.1002/mnfr.201300764

[14] Berger A, Gremaud G, Baumgartner M, Rein D, Monnard I, Kratky E, et al. Cholesterol-lowering properties of amaranth grain and oil in hamsters. International Journal for Vitamin and Nutrition Research. Feb 2003;**73**(1):39-47. DOI: 10.1024/0300-9831.73.1.39

[15] Mendonça S, Saldiva PH, Cruz RJ, Areas JAG. Amaranth protein presents cholesterol-lowering effect. Food Chemistry. July 2009;**116**(3):738-742. DOI: 10.1016/j.foodchem.2009.03.021

[16] Cherkas A, Zarkovic K, Gasparovic AC, Jaganjac M, Milkovic L, Abrahamovych O, et al. Amaranth oil reduces accumulation of 4-hydroxynonenal-histidine adducts in gastric mucosa and improves heart rate variability in duodenal peptic ulcer patients undergoing helicobacter pylori eradication. Free Radical Research. Feb 2018;**52**(2):135-149. DOI: 10.1080/10715762.2017.1418981

[17] Peter K, Gandhi P. Rediscovering the therapeutic potential of Amaranthus species: A review. Egyptian Journal of Basic and Applied Sciences. 2017;**4**:196-205. DOI: 10.1016/j.ejbas.2017.05.001

[18] Buckwheat: Wikipedia. Available from: Buckwheat - Wikipedia [Accessed: January 21, 2022]

[19] Yilmaz HO, Ayhan NY, Meric CS. Buckwheat: A useful food and its effects on human health. Current Nutrition & Food Science. Jan 2020;**16**(1):29-34. DOI: 10.2174/1573401314666180910140021

[20] Mahata D. Importance of buckwheat (Fagopyrum esculentum Moench). International Journal of Chemical Studies. 8 Aug 2018;**6**(5):2121-2125

[21] Lee CC, Hsu WH, Shen SR, Cheng YH, Wu SC. Fagopyrum tartaricum (buckwheat) improved high-glucose-induced insulin resistance in mouse hepatocytes and diabetes in fructose-rich diet-induced mice. Experimental Diabetes Research. 2012;**2012**:375673. DOI: 10.1155/2012/375673

[22] Kawa JM, Taylor CG, Przybylski R. Buckwheat concentrate reduces serum glucose in streptozotocin-diabetic rats. Journal of Agricultural and Food Chemistry. Dec 3 2003;**51**(25):7287-7291. DOI: 10.1021/jf0302153

[23] Din Z, Alam M, Ullah H, Shi D, Xu B, Li H, et al. Nutritional, phytochemical and therapeutic potential of chia seed (Salvia hispanica L.). A mini-review. Food Hydrocolloids for Health. 2021:100010. DOI: 10.1016/j.fhfh.2021.100010

[24] Ullah R, Nadeem M, Khalique A, Imran M, Mehmood S, Javid A, et al. Nutritional and therapeutic perspectives of Chia (Salvia hispanica L.): A review. Journal of Food Science and Technology. Apr 2016;**53**(4):1750-1758. DOI: 10.1007/s13197-015-1967-0

[25] Pereira E, Encina-Zelada C, Barros L, Gonzales-Barron U, Cadavez V, Ferreira ICFR. Chemical and nutritional characterization of Chenopodium quinoa Willd. (quinoa) grains: A good alternative to nutritious food. Food Chemistry. May 15 2019;**280**:110-114. DOI: 10.1016/j.foodchem.2018.12.068

[26] Motta C, Castanheira I, Gonzales GB, Delgado I, Torres D, Santos M, et al. Impact of cooking methods and malting on amino acids content in amaranth, buckwheat and quinoa. Journal of Food Composition and Analysis. 2019;**76**:58-65. DOI: 10.1016/j.jfca.2018.10.001

[27] Lejeune MP, Kovacs EM, Westerterp-Plantenga MS. Additional protein intake limits weight regain

after weight loss in humans. The British Journal of Nutrition. Feb 2005;**93**(2):281-289. DOI: 10.1079/bjn20041305

[28] Recommended Dietary Allowances: Short Report of Nutrient Requirements for Indians, Summary of Recommendations-ICMR-NIN, Hyderabad. Department of Health Research, Ministry of Health and Family Welfare; 2020. Available from: https://www.nin.res.in/RDA_short_Report_2020.html

[29] Marcinek K, Krejpcio Z. Chia seeds (Salvia Hispanica): Health promoting properties and therapeutic applications-a review. Roczniki Państwowego Zakładu Higieny. 2017;**68**(2):123-129

[30] Varli S, Sanlier N. Nutritional and health benefits of quinoa (Chenopodium quinoa wild.). Journal of Cereals Science. May 2016;**69**:371-376. DOI: 10.1016/j.jcs.2016.05.004

[31] Filho AMM, Pirozi MR, Borges JTD, SantAna MP, Chaves JBP, Coimbra JSDR. Quinoa: Nutritional, functional and Antinutritional aspects. Critical Reviews in Food Science and Nutrition. June 2015 26;**57**(8):1618-1630. DOI: 10.1080/10408398.2014.1001811

[32] Angeli V, Silva PM, Massuela DC, Khan MW, Hamar A, Khajehei F, et al. Quinoa (Chenopodium quinoa Willd.): An overview of the potentials of the "Golden grain" and socio-economic and environmental aspects of its cultivation and marketization. Food. Feb 2020;**9**:216. DOI: 10.3390/foods9020216

[33] Gawlik-Dziki U, Swieca M, Sułkowski M, Dziki D, Baraniak B, Czyz J. Antioxidant and anticancer activities of Chenopodium quinoa leaves extracts—in vitro study. Food and Chemical Toxicology. Jul 2013;**57**: 154-160. DOI: 10.1016/j.fct.2013.03.023

[34] Arts IC, Hollman PC. Polyphenols and disease risk in epidemiologic studies. The American Journal of Clinical Nutrition. Jan 2005;**81**(1 Suppl):317S-325S. DOI: 10.1093/ajcn/81.1.317S

[35] Little A, Murphy K, Solverson P. Quinoa's potential to enhance dietary Management of Obesity and Type-2 diabetes: A review of the current evidence. Diabetology. 13 May 2021;**2**(2):77-94. DOI: 10.3390/diabetology2020007

Chapter 5

Rheological Stability, Enzyme Activity, and Incorporation of Pseudocereal Powder as an Alternative Ingredient in Health-Related Food

Noorazwani Zainol, Harisun Yaakob,
Nurul Elia Aqila Abu Rahim, Nor Hasmaliana Abdul Manas,
Norsuhada Abdul Karim
and Dayang Norulfairuz Abang Zaidel

Abstract

In response to the growing recognition of health issues, people are seeking products that are inexpensive, convenient, and health-related. The incorporation of pseudocereal powder in nutraceutical sector is currently increasing because of their high nutritional profile as well as health-promoting effects. The high nutritional profile includes low starch content, high in amino acid profile, high in mineral content, and low glycemic index. Moreover, it contains high levels of phytochemicals that contain considerable amounts of flavonoids, polyphenolic chemicals, and phytosterols, making them useful in the nutraceutical sector. These bioactive compounds offer antioxidant, anti-inflammatory, and reduced risk of obesity, prediabetes, and diabetic complications. With its tremendous potential and numerous food health-related uses, pseudocereal can serve as a low-cost alternative ingredient in health-related food products. Several pseudocereal processes via enzyme activity, as well as the high rheological stability of its starch, have made pseudocereal an attractive option for modern agriculture.

Keywords: rheological stability, enzyme activity, health benefits

1. Introduction

Pseudocereal grains are edible seeds of dicotyledonous species that possess the same physical characteristics as cereal grains, such as having less or similar starch content, contribute high caloric value [1, 2] and an edible appearance [3]. The trend of pseudocereals in human diet is becoming more popular, because they fulfill high nutritional and nutraceutical needs while being gluten-free (GF). Moreover, gluten-free diet has become increasingly popular in recent years due to the increasing number of individuals having gluten intolerance, celiac disease, and self-awareness toward health. One of the topics that has received a lot of interest and is still being explored is the processing of pseudocereal powder and its application in gluten-free food development with desired texture. Pseudocereal powder manufacture has opened the door for these crops to be used into a wide range of food industries. Besides pseudocereal is an important resource for developing functional foods, research has also highlighted pseudocereal as the potential resource for health benefits [4, 5]. Secondary metabolic analysis of pseudocereals indicated that they contain considerable amounts of flavonoids family, polyphenolic components, and phytosterols, which contribute to the therapeutics properties [6–11]. In addition, they offer great potential for the future because of their high genetic diversity, allowing them to adapt to a wide range of climatic conditions, from tropical to temperate [4, 5, 12].

Pseudocereals have been referred to as twenty-first century grains due to their high nutritional value [13]. They contain high amounts of starch, fiber, and proteins with a balanced essential amino acid composition, among which are many sulfur-rich amino acids. When compared with cereals, the protein quality and quantity in pseudocereals are far superior and have emerged as a significant source of bioactive peptides in the recent decade [14]. Pseudocereal grains are rich in starch, which comprise between 60% and 80% of seed weight, which can be classified as rapidly digestible, slowly digestible, or resistant to digestion [15]. Resistant starch (RS) causes a beneficial effect on the body as it cannot be digested and absorbed in the small intestine, instead passing to the colon where it is fermented by microorganisms into short-chain fatty acids. Current dietary guidelines recommend that at least 14% RS on a total starch basis is required for health advantages. On the other hand, simple starch contains monosaccharides compound such as glucose, fructose, arabinose, xylose and disaccharides compound such as sucrose and maltose, which exist in less quantity in pseudocereal. A significant amount of dietary fiber, lipid, mineral, and vitamin contents existing in pseudocereal enhances the nutritional value of these crops and permits their entry in the functional food sector. In general, dietary fiber of pseudocereal can be divided into two groups: insoluble and soluble polysaccharides. Out of 78% of total dietary fiber content consists of insoluble polysaccharides while 22% consists of soluble polysaccharides where hemicellulose, branched-galacturonan, cellulose [4, 5] and xyloglucans, lignin, cellulose [16] are the examples of insoluble and soluble polysaccharides, respectively. For lipid profile, pseudocereal is reported to possess a high value of polyunsaturated fatty acid, which consists of linolenic acid and linoleic acid [17, 18] whereby unsaturated fatty acid, oleic acid, and palmitic acid are among the abundant fatty acids existing [19, 20]. The mineral compounds of pseudocereal are abundant in coat; therefore, as a whole pseudocereal are a good source of mineral.

2. The rheological modification of pseudocereal starches

The study of starch gelatinization properties through viscometer analysis is very important for understanding the viscosity changes and evaluating the disintegration of starch components and their tendency to regenerate when forming new hydrogen bonds, thereby forming viscoelastic gels [21]. The pasting properties of native pseudocereal starches are summarized in **Table 1**. From **Table 1**, the measurements of pseudocereal starch paste's viscosity are analyzed using Modular Compact Rheometer (unit recorded as cP), Rapid Visco-Analyzer (RVA), Brabender Amylograph (BA),

Native pseudocereal starch	Viscosity (^{a}cP/^{b}mPa s/^{c}RVU/^{d}BU)*					Pasting temperature (°C)	Pasting time (min)
	Peak	Trough	Breakdown	Final	Setback		
Amaranth—*Amaranthus hypochondriacus*	2176^{a}	1533^{a}	643^{a}	1710^{a}	177^{a}	72	3.95
– *A. caudatus*	2285.85^{b}	—	1247.15^{b}	1276.7^{b}	262.64^{b}	64.32	5.13
– *Amaranthus* sp.	73.42^{c}	—	13.5^{c}	68.54^{c}	8.63^{c}	81.88	—
Buckwheat	3133^{a}	1650^{a}	—	3912^{a}	—	—	—
	4019^{a}	—	1641^{a}	4293^{a}	1915^{a}	63.7	—
	4589^{a}	2171^{a}	2418^{a}	3986^{a}	1816^{a}	68.75	3.47
	600^{d}	—	1220^{d}	—	620^{d}	—	—
Quinoa	101.08^{c}	—	−0.86^{c}	114.39^{c}	12.44^{c}	95	—

**cP: centipoise; mPa s: millipascal-second; RVU: Rapid Viscosity Unit, BU: Brabender Unit.*

Table 1.
Pasting properties of native pseudocereal starches.

or using a dynamic rheometer in a flow temperature ramp mode. In general, data obtained as in **Table 1** show that the pasting temperature affects the ability of starch to imbibe water whereby as the pasting temperature rises, the likelihood of paste creation rises. Hence, it can be suggested that in the presence of water and heat, starch granules swell and form paste by imbibing water [21]. The pasting temperature of pseudocereal starch as in **Table 1** ranges from 63.7 to 95°C, and it can be differentiated into two groups, which is the higher pasting temperature ranging from 81.88–95°C [22, 23] while the lower pasting temperature ranges from 63.7 to 68.75°C [21, 24, 25]. The pasting temperature depends on the size of the starch granules where small granules are more resistant to rupture and loss of molecular order, so this might explain the relatively high pasting temperature [26].

The modifications of pseudocereal starches were studied by many researchers to improve the functional and rheological properties of pseudocereal starch [22–25, 27]. Pasting properties of modified pseudocereal starches in comparison with their respective native pseudocereal starches are summarized in **Table 2**. There are three types of modified pseudocereal, namely physical modification, chemical modification, and physicochemical modification as in **Table 2**. In general, chemical modification of starch resulted in significantly increased peak viscosity compared with the other two types of modified pseudocereal. This is probably due to the increased granular stiffness, which is resultant of starch chain interactions within the amorphous region and an increase in crystalline order [24]. Oxidization, acetylation, and octenylsuccinylated (OSA) as in **Table 2** increased the peak viscosity of *Amaranthus hypochondriacus* that might be accredited to the higher swelling power and comparable solubility of starch relative to native starch. Final viscosity signifies the starch ability to develop viscous paste on cooling after cooking the starch solution.

Physical modifications of pseudocereal starches by heat moisture treatment (HMT) were studied in two types of amaranth spp. such as *A. caudatus* [21] and *A. hypochondriacus* [22] as in **Table 2**. Heat moisture treatment causes intensifying decrement in setback viscosity with rising amylose content in starches as high-temperature treatment supports added interactions between amylose-amylose and

Type of starch modification	Type of pseudocereal starches	Pasting properties						
		viscosity					Pasting temp.	Pasting time
		Peak	Trough	Breakdown	Final	Setback		
Chemical modification								
1) Oxidation	Amaranth (*Amaranthus hypochondriacus*)	↑	↑	↑	↑	↑	↓	↓
2) Acetylation	Amaranth (*A. hypochondriacus*)	↑	↓	↑	↓	↑	↓	↓
	Buckwheat	↑	—	↓		↓	—	—
3) Alcoholic-Alkali Treatment	Buckwheat	↓	↓	↓	↑	↑	↓	↑
4) Octenylsuccinylated (OSA)	Amaranth (*Amaranthus* sp.)	↑	—	↑	↑	↑	↓	—
	Quinoa	↑	—	↑	↑	↑	↓	—
Physical modification								
1) Annealing	Buckwheat	↓	—	↓	↓	↓	↑	—
2) Heat-Moisture Treatment (HMT): 85 °C	Amaranth (*A. hypochondriacus*)	↑	↓	↑	↓	↑	↑	↑
: 00°C	Amaranth (*A. hypochondriacus*)	↑	↓	↑	↓	↑	↑	↓
: 20 °C	Amaranth (*A. hypochondriacus*)	↑	↑	↑	↑	↑	↑	↑
3) HMT at 120°C(15 min): 10% moisture	Amaranth (*A. caudatus*)	↓	—	↓	↑	↑	↓	↓
: 15% moisture	Amaranth (*A. caudatus*)	↓	—	↓	↑	↓	↑	↓
: 20% moisture	Amaranth (*A. caudatus*)	↓	—	↑	↓		↑	↑
(30 min): 10% moisture	Amaranth (*A. caudatus*)	↑	—	↑	↑	↑	↓	↓
: 15% moisture	Amaranth (*A. caudatus*)	↓	—	↓	↓	↓	↑	↓
: 20% moisture	Amaranth (*A. caudatus*)	↓	—	↓	↓	↓	↑	↑
(60 min): 10% moisture	Amaranth (*A. caudatus*)	↓	—	↓	↑	↑	↓	↓

Type of starch modification	Type of pseudocereal starches	Pasting properties						
		viscosity					Pasting temp.	Pasting time
		Peak	Trough	Breakdown	Final	Setback		
: 15% moisture	Amaranth (*A. caudatus*)	↓	—	↓	↓	↓	↑	↓
: 20% moisture	Amaranth (*A. caudatus*)	↓	—	↓	↓	↓	↑	↑
4) HMT at 110°C: 20% moisture	Buckwheat	↓	—	↓	↓	↑	↑	—
: 25% moisture	Buckwheat	↓	—	↓	↓	↑	↑	—
: 30% moisture	Buckwheat	↓	—	↓	↓	↑	↑	—
: 35% moisture	Buckwheat	↓	—	↓	↓	↓	↑	—
5) Ball Milling Treatment	Buckwheat	↓	↓	↓	↓	↓	↓	↑
6 Drum Drying	Buckwheat	↑	↓	↑	↓	↑	↓	↓
Physico-chemical modification								
Acid hydrolysis + HMT	Buckwheat	↓	↑	—	↑	—	—	—

Table 2.
Pasting properties of modified pseudocereal starches in comparison with the native starches (refer ***Table 1****).*

amylopectin-amylopectin chains that lessen amylase leaching and decrease setback viscosity. From **Table 2**, it can be observed that all HMT of modified-amaranth (*A. caudatus*) starches and modified-buckwheat starches decreases in peak viscosity and breakdown viscosity as compared with native starch. It indicates that the modified starches are more stable as compared with native one. Meanwhile, Sindhu and his team [22] found the contradict results, which increase in peak, breakdown, and setback viscosity that reflects the poor stability of modified starches and starch retrogradation occurred. All physical treatments aim to modify the granular structure of native starch and convert it to cold-dissolvable starch or crystallization of starch.

The hydrothermal treatment of native starch reduced its ultimate viscosity at lower temperatures (85 and 100°C), but increased it significantly at higher temperatures (120°C). The eventual viscosity of all starch samples was lower than the peak viscosity, which could be due to some glycosidic linkage breakdown. In addition to the breakdown viscosity, the stability of starch pastes is determined by their breaking point, and higher breaking point values indicate inferior stability during continuous heating and shearing procedures in comparison to native starch. Except for acetylated starch, which showed a nonsignificant rise in setback viscosity when compared with native starch, all treated starches showed a substantial increase in setback viscosity. The largest setback viscosity was found in oxidized starch, and results from a freeze-thaw stability experiment confirmed this. Oxidized starch had the highest syneresis, while acetylated starch had the lowest. The setback viscosity varies depending on the amount of amylose leaching, the size of the granules, and the type of swelling granules. In this study, modified starch samples had an enhanced setback viscosity due to the waxy and low amylose characteristics of the amaranth starch used. Increases in pasting temperatures of heat-moisture-treated starches indicated that amylopectin chain connections were strengthening and interactions between them expanding. Starch pastes were statistically significantly reduced in pasting temperature and peak time as a result of acetylation and oxidation processes. Because the insertion of functional groups modulated the amorphous region and decreased the intermolecular hydrogen bonds, the pasting temperature of the starch granules was lower. Modification improves the application of modified starch in products where the thickening ingredient must gelatinize quickly at low temperatures by lowering the pasting temperature and peak time. The increased efficiency of such items also decreases the energy costs involved in their processing. As a consequence, acetylated and oxidized starches are usable in formulations that require low-temperature cooking/processing to obtain pastes [22, 28].

The effect of octenyl succinylation on the functional characteristics of *Amaranthus paniculatus* starch was investigated by Bhosale and Singhal [29]. The swelling power, paste clarity, freeze-thaw stability, enhanced viscosity, and lowered gelatinization temperature of OSA-modified amaranth starch were all improved. These findings suggest that OSA-modified amaranth starch could have applications in the food business, particularly in emulsification. Pal et al. [30] investigated the qualities of hydroxypropyl derivatives derived from *A. paniculatus* starch and discovered a considerable improvement in freeze-thaw stability, suggesting that it could be used as a thickening agent in frozen foods. All starches (amaranth/quinoa) had increased pasting viscosities following modification of octenylsuccinylate (OSA), but RVA profiles were affected in different ways. In contrast to native starches, OSA starches were found to paste at a lower temperature between 73.7 and 81.4°C. Due to the fact that OSA starches have loosely packed surface areas, resulting in lower pasting temperatures, the OSA group produces spatial hindrance, which is responsible for weakening internal hydrogen bonds, which increases water absorption and lowers energy expenditure for gelatinization [23]. There might be additional influences on PT change from starch compositional aspects, such as the chain length of amylopectin, granule surface, and packing arrangement within the granules. As a result of the substitution of OSA on starch granules, the pasting qualities are also compromised. Peak viscosity can be defined as the water-holding capacity of starch granules in terms of swelling and shearing ability. Starches with high peak viscosity are suited for application as food thickeners, while a low percentage of OSA starch can replace higher levels of unmodified starch. Amylose content and long-chain fraction of amylopectin have been reported as major factors influencing peak viscosity [23, 24]. Modification of quinoa starch with OSA showed that a substitution degree of 3.21% is optimal for emulsifier formation and stabilization. A higher degree of substitution (4.66%) results in the aggregation of starch granules and the decrease of starch granule stable emulsion. In addition, OSA modification is more effective than heat treatment in providing hydrophobic characteristics to quinoa. The heat treatment is only slightly better than the natural starch granules [31].

Several studies have been reported about different physical modification methods in buckwheat starches, some of these are roasting process [32], microwave and annealing treatments [33], drum-drying and ball-milling treatment [24] high-pressure and high-temperature treatment [34], heat moisture treatment and annealing [24], hydrothermal processing [35], autoclaving/cooling [36], and others. The duration and quality of the gelatinization process as well as the viscosity and behavior of the gelatinization also change in nearly identical ways, including decreased or increased pasting viscosity, increased or decreased swelling power and solubility, increased retrograded starch content, increased gelatinization temperature, and slower digestion of the gelatinization [37].

3. Application of enzyme in pseudocereals

Enzymes are necessary for the production of compounds from grains that are used in contemporary foods and beverages. Enzymes have been identified as having the ability to improve the processing behavior or qualities of cereal and pseudocereals meals such as flavor, texture, and shelf-life with minimal impact on nutritional content [38].

Grain contains endogenous and exogenous enzymes. Endogenous enzymes are found naturally in grain kernels and are primarily found in the outer layer, fiber, and bacteria. Meanwhile, exogenous enzymes are created by bacteria on the surface. These enzymes influence grain raw materials quality and processing properties, mainly when humidity and time are present. Some enzymes are found in cereals, are frequently of microbial origin, and are given as pretreatment and manufacturing agents. Enzymes can contribute significantly by increasing the usage of raw materials and improving the impact of food and beverages [39]. **Table 3** shows the benefits of exogenous and endogenous enzymes in the diet. In general, both exogenous and endogenous enzymes influence the quality of the pseudocereal grains as listed in **Table 3** below. Apparently, the existence of endogenous enzyme gives a huge impact on the physical-chemical properties of pseudocereal grain compared with exogenous enzyme.

Exogenous enzymes	Endogenous enzymes
• To boost the nutritional value • Modify and improve nutritional quality by allowing starch and non-starch components to interact. • Microbial origin • Reducing the availability of digestive enzymes and, as a result, the pace of starch digestion	• Reducing the availability of digestive enzymes and, as a result, the pace of starch digestion • Increase nutritional value and palatability by manipulating the main biological macromolecules, such as carbohydrates, lipids, proteins, nucleic acids, and simple molecules such as vitamins, amino acids, and sugars. • Catalyzing natural reaction during germination and sprouting • Provides taste to the mix, which affects sensory characteristics • Involve the grain's raw material's quality and processing qualities • Deteriorate the processing characteristics of flour and other grain products • Capable of altering cereal structure and functional qualities

Table 3.
The advantages of exogenous and endogenous enzymes in food [38, 40, 41].

The areas of enzyme in grain processing are pervasive in terms of raw material and enzyme-catalyzed processes. The most important contemporary sectors involving enzyme treatment of grains are energy supply, bioethanol, biomaterials, digestible films, and sustainable biomass utilization. The enzymes work with polysaccharides and proteins to control and use starch structure, which is significant in the food and beverage industries [42].

3.1 The involvement of enzymes in seed germination

Seed germination is a phenomenon governed by various mechanisms required to transform a seed into a new plant. The mature seed includes the necessary components to participate in the processes that control germination, including the enzymes that will aid in the process. Germination demonstrates the nutritional value and availability of proteins and amino acids while decreasing the amount of anti-nutritive substances [43]. Enzymes help restore broken DNA during the drying and germination of the grain, resulting in proper seedling growth.

Unrefined cereal crops need a variety of pretreatment processes, including the use of enzymes in addition to standard techniques. By altering the molecular structure and the amount and quality of nutrients, phytochemicals, and harmful compounds, enzyme pretreatment improves processability, safety, stability, or technical and nutritional utility [43]. For example, enzymes can reduce mycotoxin levels by biotransforming mycotoxin into harmless metabolites [38].

Research demonstrated that enzymatic mycotoxin destruction depends on the enzyme-producing source, its concentration, and the circumstances used [44]. Susanna and Prabhasankar [45] developed an outstanding quality hypoimmunogenic pasta using a blend of xylanase, protease, and transglutaminase, which might be a gluten-free alternative [45, 46] and showed the use of enzymes in cereal grain polishing. Depolymerization of bran carbohydrates happens due to cell wall degrading enzymes in this process, altering phenolic mobilization and dietary fiber solubilization. Carbohydrate-cleaving enzymes, such as cellulases (e.g., endoglucanase, exoglycanases, and beta-glucosidase), xylanases, glucanases, and esterases, undertake enzyme biopolishing [46]. **Table 4** shows the enzymes utilized and the progress

Substances	Enzymes	Improvement
Nutrition's level	• Hemicellulases	Soluble dietary content is increased
Quality	• Amylases • Proteases • Glucose oxidases • Hemicellulases • Lipoxygenases	Balancing the change of recipe, replacement of potassium bromates, sodium metabisulfite, emulsifier, vital gluten, and fat baking reduction
Taste	• Amylases • Proteases • Lipoxygenases • Lipases • Glucose oxidases	Fermentation substrates production and aroma precursors
Color	• Amylases • Hemicellulases • Lipoxygenases	Brownish, crust color improvement and bleaching effects
Surface structure	• Hemicellulases • Amylases • Proteases • Lipases	Smoother particles,
Strength	• Amylases • Hemicellulases	Freshen up, anti-evaporate, longer life span
Size/volume	• Amylases • Hemicellulases • Cellulases • Lipases	Larger size/volume

Table 4.
The types of enzymes used and the improvement toward pseudocereals [38].

toward pseudocereals. In general, these enzymes have been used in improving nutrition level, quality, taste, color, surface structure, strength, and size. Apparently, amylases and hemicellulase are the two enzymes that are important for pseudocereal improvement. The taste and quality of pseudocereal as shown in **Table 4** were affected by the same group of enzymes, namely amylases, proteases, glucose oxidases, hemicellulases, and lipoxygenases.

3.2 Fermentation in pseudocereal processing

Fermentation is an ancient and cost-effective way of generating and storing foods that may be applied to grain processing. Fermentation is the process that releases energy by oxidizing carbohydrates without the need of an external electron acceptor. Most of the time, enzymes are required in the fermentation process to speed up the reaction. For example, alcohol cannot be produced without the enzyme amylase, which breaks down starch into simple sugar. Moreover, fermentation is impossible without enzymes. Fermentation is one of the oldest and most cost-effective methods of food preservation and processing. Due to the enzymatic degradation of antinutritional compounds such as phytate, fermentation enhances the availability of particular amino acids, B vitamins, and minerals, including iron, zinc, and calcium [42]. Certain antinutrient substances in pseudocereals such as phytic acid, polyphenols, and protein inhibitors could negatively impact on malnutritions [47]. Fermentation with Lactic Acid Bacteria (LAB) can increase pseudocereals' nutritional and functional qualities [48].

Cereal and pseudocereal fermentation is critical in the creation of chemicals that have a significant impact on organoleptic features such as scent, taste, and texture as well as the enhancement of nutritional values, all of which have a good impact on human health [47]. Microorganisms may be found in practically every biological niche; cereals and pseudocereals generally provide an excellent substrate for microbial fermentations. Polysaccharides are abundant, which microorganisms may use as a carbon and energy source during fermentation. Fermented items made from common cereals and pseudocereals are ubiquitous worldwide [48]. LAB, enterobacteria, aerobic spore formers, and other microbiota fighting for resources are typical in cereal and pseudocereal grains. The pH value, water activity, salt concentration, temperature, and food matrix composition all influence the kind of bacteria present in each fermented meal [48].

4. Functional and health benefit offered by pseudocereal

Approximately 80% of the human diet is composed of cereals such as corn, wheat, and rice. These grains are biofortified in order to boost vitamin and other essential micronutrient levels. However, pseudocereals, which are naturally enriched with a lot of essential micronutrients and nutraceutical ingredients, are not well utilized for its functional and health benefits to the human.

Pseudocereals are a novelty in human diets as they are gluten-free (GF) grains with a high nutritional and nutraceutical value. Additionally, recent research suggests that pseudo cereals may have health benefits, placing these crops in the role of important resources for the development of functional foods [4]. Protein quality and quantity in pseudo cereals are considerably superior to cereal quality and quantity, so they can be considered functional foods. In addition to amino acids such as arginine, tryptophan, lysine, and histidine, pseudocereals are rich in essential amino acids for infant and child nutrition, rendering them useful as food supplements. Protein nutritional quality can be measured using several parameters including protein efficiency ratio (PER) or net protein use (NPU), digestibility and bioavailability of protein, and availability of lysine. Pseudo cereal protein levels are thus larger than cereal protein levels and comparable to casein levels. Proteins of pseudo cereals are similar to those of legumes, since they have 2S albumin, 11S globulin, and 7S globulin. Furthermore, pseudocereal proteins are acceptable for celiac disease patients due to their low prolamine level [49].

Buckwheat is gaining popularity as a potential functional food due to its health-promoting components such as phenolic compounds and sterols. It is a good source of protein, dietary fiber, fat, and minerals [50]. Foods that give specific health benefits (health claims) exceeding their nutritional worth are referred to as functional foods, although their intake is not required for humankind [51]. Several biological and health benefits can be attributed to the consumption of buckwheat and buckwheat products, including hypocholesterolemic, hypoglycemic, anticancer, and anti-inflammatory properties. These health benefits are said to be, at least in part, attributed to buckwheat proteins and phenolic compounds [52]. Some of these health advantages may be due to the antioxidant activity of these compounds, but recently identified mechanisms of action may also be related [53, 54]. Despite pseudocereals' composition and properties, there are still relatively little *in vivo* studies and limited human trials supporting its functional benefit. Most studies have linked consumption of pseudocereals or their bioactive components to a protective effect against obesity, prediabetes, and diabetes complications. Thus, the rat plasma ghrelin levels were reduced while postprandial leptin and cholecystokinin levels increased after consuming amaranth-protein-based diets [55]. Amaranth protein also modulates the microbiota composition of mice with obesity induced by diet [56]. In addition, a streptozotocin-induced diabetes model revealed that amaranth protein improved glucose tolerance and boosted plasma insulin levels [57]. In Wistar rats and spontaneously hypertensive rats, protein hydrolyzates showed significant antithrombotic effects [58] and antihypertensive [59].

For 6 weeks, rats fed with high-fat diet showed a lowering of cholesterol and a reduction of inflammation caused by tartary buckwheat protein, as well as changes in the animals' microbiota [60]. In obese diabetic mice [61] and Wistar rats [62], quinoa intake prevented hyperglycemia, decreased total cholesterol, and decreased LDL cholesterol. Recent research has demonstrated that quinoa can also modulate inflammatory biomarkers in the liver as well as dwindle hepatic steatosis and cholesterol accumulation. Furthermore, there has been evidence that quinoa phytoecdysteroid-enriched extracts reduce adipose tissue, regulate gene expressions involved in fat storage, and attenuate inflammation and insulin resistance in a mouse model with diet-induced obesity [63]. The scientists also found an increase in glucose oxidation and fecal lipid discharge without influencing stool sizes, in addition to an increase in energy expenditure without modifying food consumption or activity [64].

Until recently, there have been relatively few human studies evaluating the benefits of pseudocereals. Ruales et al. [65] mentioned that two times a day administration of 100g of quinoa to 50–65-month-old boys living in low-income Ecuador increases plasma insulin-like growth factor (IGF-1). Therefore, quinoa-enriched baby food is able to prevent child malnutrition by providing sufficient protein and other essential nutrients. Additionally, supplementation of the diet with quinoa has shown to impact cardiovascular and metabolic parameters in both healthy [66] and overweight and obese people [53, 67, 68].

5. Conclusions

Various fields of study are currently being conducted, from its functional and rheological properties as well as enzyme immobilization and its application. Pseudocereal is suitable for use in a wide variety of food applications since it is packed with nutrients, consists of promising health benefits promoter, and is a source of energy. Furthermore, ongoing research into rheological modification of resistant starch could offer a number of possibilities and make it a possible source for use in the food sector, resulting in a substantial impact on food sustainability. Although research on the substances obtained from pseudocereal could be conducted, safety factors should be addressed in order to develop health-related food products.

Conflict of interest

The authors declare no conflict of interest.

Nomenclature

Gluten-free	GF
Rapid Visco-Analyzer	RVA
Brabender Amylograph	BA
Octenylsuccinylate	OSA
Heat moisture treatment	HMT
Lactic Acid Bacteria	LAB
Protein efficiency ratio	PER
Net protein use	NPU
Insulin-like growth factor	IGF-1

Author details

Noorazwani Zainol[1*], Harisun Yaakob[1], Nurul Elia Aqila Abu Rahim[2], Nor Hasmaliana Abdul Manas[1,2], Norsuhada Abdul Karim[2] and Dayang Norulfairuz Abang Zaidel[1,2]

1 Institute of Bioproduct Development, Universiti Teknologi Malaysia, Johor Bahru, Malaysia

2 Food and Biomaterial Engineering Research Group, School of Chemical and Energy Engineering, Universiti Teknologi Malaysia, Johor Bahru, Malaysia

*Address all correspondence to: azwani@ibd.utm.my

References

[1] Kreft I, Zhou M, Golob A, Germ M, Likar M, Dziedzic K, et al. Breeding buckwheat for nutritional quality. Breeding Science. 2020;**70**:67-73

[2] Valdivia-Lopez MA, Tecante A. Chia (*Salvia hispanica*): A review of native Mexican seed and its nutritional and functional properties. Advances in Food and Nutrition Research. 2015;**75**:53-75

[3] Alvarez-Jubete L, Arendt EK, Gallagher E. Nutritive value of pseudocereals and their increasing use as functional gluten-free ingredients. Trends in Food Science & Technology. 2010;**21**:106-113. DOI: 10.1016/j.tifs.2009.10.014

[4] Joshi DC, Sood S, Hosahatti R, Kant L, Pattanayak A, Kumar A, et al. From zero to hero: The past, present and future of grain amaranth breeding. Theoretical and Applied Genetics. 2018;**131**:1807-1823. DOI: 10.1007/s00122-018-3138-y

[5] Joshi DC, Chaudhari GV, Sood S, Kant L, Pattanayak A, Zhang K, et al. Revisiting the versatile buckwheat: Reinvigorating genetic gains through integrated breeding and genomics approach. Planta. 2019;**250**:783-801. DOI: 10.1007/s00425-018-03080-4

[6] Gebremariam MM, Zarnkow M, Becker T. Teff (Eragrostistef) as a raw material for malting, brewing and manufacturing of gluten-free foods and beverages: A review. Journal of Food Science and Technology. 2014;**51**:2881-2895

[7] Martínez-Cruz O, Paredes-Lopez O. Phytochemical pro file and nutraceutical potential of chia seeds (*Salvia hispanica* L.) by ultra-high performance liquid chromatography. Journal of Chromatography A. 2014;**1346**:43-48

[8] Zhang L, Liu R, Niu W. Phytochemical and anti-proliferative activity of proso millet. PLoS One. 2014;**9**:e104058

[9] Tang Y, Tsao R. Phytochemicals in quinoa and amaranth grains and their antioxidant, anti-inflammatory and potential health beneficial effects: A review. Molecular Nutrition & Food Research. 2017;**61**:1600767

[10] Dar FA, Pirzadah TB, Malik B, Tahir I, Rehman RU. Molecular genetics of buckwheat and its role in crop improvement. In: Zhou M, Kreft I, Tang Y, Suvorova G, editors. Buckwheat Germplasm in the World. Istedn: Elsevier Publications USA; 2018. pp. 271-286

[11] Pirzadah TB, Malik B, Tahir I, Qureshi MI, Rehman RU. Characterization of mercury-induced stress biomarkers in *Fagopyrum tataricum* plants. International Journal of Phytoremediation. 2018;**20**(3):225-236

[12] Ruiz KB et al. Quinoa diversity and sustainability for food security under climate change. Agronomy for Sustainable Development. 2013;**34**:349-359. DOI: 10.1007/s13593-013-0195-0

[13] FAO. Food and Agriculture Organization Regional Office for Latin America, and the Caribbean PROINPA. Quinoa: An Ancient Crop to Contribute to World Food Security. Santiago: FAO Regional Office for Latin American and the Caribbean; 2011. Available from: http://www.fao.org/alc/file/media/pubs/2011/cultivo_quinua_en.Pdf

[14] Mendonça S et al. Amaranth protein presents cholesterol-lowering effect. Food Chemistry. 2009;**116**:738-742. DOI: 10.1016/j.foodchem.2009.03.021

[15] Lockyer S, Nugent AP. Health effects of resistant starch. Nutrition Bulletin. 2017;**42**:10-41. DOI: 10.1111/nbu.12244

[16] Dziedzic K et al. Influence of technological process during buckwheat groats production on dietary fibre content and sorption of bile acids. Food Research International. 2012;**47**:279-283. DOI: 10.1016/j.foodres.2011.07.020

[17] Pachari-Vera E et al. Comparison of the lipid profile and tocopherol content of four Peruvian quinoa (Chenopodium quinoa Willd.) cultivars ('Amarilla de Maranganí', 'Blanca de Juli', INIA 415 'Roja Pasankalla', INIA 420 'Negra Collana') during germination. Journal of Cereal Science. 2019;**88**:132-137. DOI: 10.1016/j.jcs.2019.05.015.2019

[18] Tang Y et al. Assessing the fatty acid composition, carotenoid, and tocopherol compositions of amaranth and quinoa seeds grown in Ontario and their overall contribution to nutritional quality. Journal of Agricultural and Food Chemistry. 2016;**64**:1103-1110. DOI: 10.1021/acs.jafc.5b05414

[19] Pereira E et al. Chemical and nutritional characterization of *Chenopodium quinoa* Willd. (quinoa) grains: A good alternative to nutritious food. Food Chemistry. 2019;**280**:110-114. DOI: 10.1016/j.foodchem.2018.12.068

[20] Shukla A et al. Genetic diversity analysis in buckwheat germplasm for nutritional traits. Indian Journal of Experimental Biology. 2018;**56**:827-837. Available from: http://nopr.niscair.res.in/handle/123456789/45342

[21] Bet CD, de Oliveira CS, Colman TAD, Marinho MT, Lacerda LG, Ramos AP, et al. Organic amaranth starch: A study of its technological properties after heat-moisture treatment. Food Chemistry. 2018;**264**:435-442

[22] Sindhu R, Devi A, Khatkar BS. Morphology, structure and functionality of acetylated, oxidized and heat moisture treated amaranth starches. Food Hydrocolloids. 2021;**118**(106800):1-10

[23] Wen Y, Yao T, Xu Y, Corke H, Sui Z. Pasting, thermal and rheological properties of octenylsuccinylate modified starches from diverse small granule starches differing in amylose content. Journal of Cereal Science. 2020;**95**(103030):1-7

[24] Li W, Cao F, Fan J, Ouyang S, Luo Q, Zheng J, et al. Physically modified common buckwheat starch and their physicochemical and structural properties. Food Hydrocolloids. 2014;**40**:237-244

[25] Liu H, Guo X, Li W, Wang X, Lv M, Peng Q, et al. Changes in physicochemical properties and in vitro digestibility of common buckwheat starch by heat-moisture treatment and annealing. Carbohydrate Polymers. 2015;**132**:237-244

[26] Akanbi TO, Nazamid S, Adebowale AA. Functional and pasting properties of a tropical breadfruit (*Artocarpus altilis*) starch from Ile-Ife, Osun State, Nigeria. International Food Research Journal. 2009;**16**:151-157

[27] Zheng GH, Sosulski FW, Tyler RT. Wet-milling, composition and functional properties of starch and protein isolated from buckwheat groats. Food Research International. 1997;**30**:493-502

[28] Malik MA, Saxena DC. Effect on physicochemical and thermal properties of buckwheat (*Fagopyrum esculentum*) starch by acid hydrolysis combined with heat moisture treatment. Journal of Food Processing and Preservation. 2016;**40**(6):1-12

[29] Bhosale R, Singhal R. Effect of octenylsuccinylation on physicochemical and functional properties of waxy maize and amaranth starches. Carbohydrate Polymers. 2007;**68**:447-456

[30] Pal J, Singhal RS, Kulkarni PR. Physicochemical properties of hydroxypropyl derivative from corn and amaranth starch. Carbohydrate Polymers. 2002;**48**:49-53

[31] Rayner M, Sjöö M, Timgren A, Dejmek P. Quinoa starch granules as stabilizing particles for production of Pickering emulsions. Faraday Discussions. 2012;**158**:139-155

[32] Christa K, Soral-Śmietana M, Lewandowicz G. Buckwheat starch: Structure, functionality and enzyme *in vitro* susceptibility upon the roasting process. International Journal of Food Sciences and Nutrition. 2009;**60**:140-154

[33] Gupta M, Gill BS, Bawa AS. Gelatinization and X-ray crystallography of buckwheat starch: Effect of microwave and annealing treatments. International Journal of Food Properties. 2008;**11**:173-185

[34] Vallons KJR, Arendt EK. Effects of high pressure and temperature on buckwheat starch characteristics. European Food Research and Technology. 2009;**230**:343-351

[35] Skrabanja V, Kreft I. Resistant starch formation following autoclaving of buckwheat (*Fagopyrum esculentum* Moench) groats. An in vitro study. Journal of Agricultural and Food Chemistry. 1998;**46**:2020-2023

[36] Skrabanja V, Laerke HN, Kreft I. Effects of hydrothermal processing of buckwheat (*Fagopyrum esculentum* Moench) groats on starch enzymatic availability *in vitro* and *in vivo* in rats. Journal of Cereal Science. 1998;**28**:209-214

[37] Perez-Rea D, Antezana-Gomez R. Chapter 12- The functionality of pseudocereal starches. In: Sjöö M, Nilsson L, editors. Starch in Food Structure, Function and Applications. 2nd ed. United Kingdom: Woodhead Publishing Series in Food Science, Technology and Nutrition (Elsevier); 2018. pp. 509-542

[38] Sasthri VM, Krishnakumar N, Prabhasankar P. Advances in conventional cereal and pseudocereal processing. In: Pojić M, Tiwari U, editors. Innovative Processing Technologies for Healthy Grains. John Wiley & Sons; 30 Dec 2020. pp. 61-81. DOI: 10.1002/97811194 70182.ch4

[39] Chapman J, E.Ismail A, Zoica Dinu C. Industrial Applications of Enzyme: Recent Advance, Techniques and Outlook. Catalysts. 2018;**8**:238. DOI: 10.3390/catal8060238

[40] Kerpes R, Fischer S, Becker T. The production of gluten-free beer: Degradation of hordeins during malting and brewing and the application of modern process technology focusing on endogenous malt peptidases. Trends in Food Science and Technology. 2017;**67**:129-138. DOI: 10.1016/j.tifs.2017.07.004

[41] Mir NA, Riar CS, Singh S. Nutritional constituents of pseudocereals and their potential use in food systems: A review. Trends in Food Science and Technology. 2018;**75**(March):170-180. DOI: 10.1016/j.tifs.2018.03.016

[42] Berezina NA, Nikitin IA, Khmeleva EV, Glebova NV, Makarova NA. Features of technological characteristics of cereal and pseudocereal

flour. BIO Web of Conferences. 2020;**17**:00121. DOI: 10.1051/bioconf/20201700121

[43] Muñoz-Llandes CR, Fabiola Araceli Guzmán-Ortiz FA, Román-Gutiérrez AD, Patricia López-Perea P, Castro-Rosas J, Vargas-Torres A. Effect of germination on antinutritional compounds of grains and seeds. In: Mora- Escobedo R, Martinez C, et al, editors. Germination: Types, Process and Effects. New York: Nova Science Publisher; pp. 83-100. ISBN: 978-1-53615-973-8. Available from: https://www.researchgate.net/publication/348521057_Effect_of_Germination_on_Antinutritional_Compounds_of_Grains_and_Seeds

[44] Loi M, Fanelli F, Liuzzi VC, Logrieco AF, Mulè G. Mycotoxin biotransformation by native and commercial enzymes: Present and future perspectives. Toxins. 2017;**9**(4):111. DOI: 10.3390/toxins9040111

[45] Susanna S, Prabhasankar P. Effect of different enzymes on immunogenicity of pasta. Food and Agricultural Immunology. 2015;**26**(2):231-247. DOI: 10.1080/09540105.2014.893999

[46] Singh A, Karmakar S, Jacob BS, Bhattacharya P, Kumar SPJ, Banerjee R. Enzymatic polishing of cereal grains for improved nutrient retainment. Journal of Food Science and Technology. 2015;**52**(6):3147-3157. DOI: 10.1007/s13197-014-1405-8

[47] Pirzadah TB, Malik B. Pseudocereals as super foods of 21st century: Recent technological interventions. Journal of Agriculture and Food Research. 2020;**2**(May):100052. DOI: 10.1016/j.jafr.2020.100052

[48] Rollán GC, Gerez CL, Leblanc JG. Lactic fermentation as a strategy to improve the nutritional and functional values of pseudocereals. Frontiers in Nutrition. 2019;**6**(July):98. DOI: 10.3389/fnut.2019.00098

[49] Świeca M, Regula J, Suliburska J, Zlotek U, Gawlik-Dziki U, Ferreira IM. Safeness of diets based on gluten-free buckwheat bread enriched with seeds and nuts—Effect on oxidative and biochemical parameters in rat serum. Nutrients. 2020;**12**(1):41

[50] Krkošková B, Mrazova Z. Prophylactic components of buckwheat. Food Research International. 2005; **38**(5):561-568

[51] González-Sarrías A, Larrosa M, García-Conesa MT, Tomás-Barberán FA, Espín JC. Nutraceuticals for older people: Facts, fictions and gaps in knowledge. Maturitas. 2013;**75**(4):313-334

[52] Zhang ZL, Zhou ML, Tang Y, Li FL, Tang YX, Shao JR, et al. Bioactive compounds in functional buckwheat food. Food Research International. 2012;**49**(1):389-395

[53] Liu RH. Health benefits of fruit and vegetables are from additive and synergistic combinations of phytochemicals. The American Journal of Clinical Nutrition. 2003;**78**(3):517S-520S

[54] D'Archivio M, Filesi C, Varì R, Scazzocchio B, Masella R. Bioavailability of the polyphenols: Status and controversies. International Journal of Molecular Sciences. 2010;**11**(4):1321-1342

[55] Mithila MV, Khanum F. Effectual comparison of quinoa and amaranth supplemented diets in controlling appetite; a biochemical study in rats. Journal of Food Science and Technology. 2015;**52**(10):6735-6741

[56] Olguín-Calderón D, González-Escobar JL, Ríos-Villa R, Dibildox-Alvarado E, Leon-Rodriguez D,

de la Rosa APB. Modulation of caecal microbiome in obese mice associated with administration of amaranth or soybean protein isolates. Polish Journal of Food and Nutrition Sciences. 2019;**69**(19(1):35-44

[57] Jorge SS, Raúl RB, Isabel GL, Edith PA, Bernardo EB, César AP, et al. Dipeptidyl peptidase IV inhibitory activity of protein hydrolyzates from *Amaranthus hypochondriacus* L. Grain and their influence on postprandial glycemia in Streptozotocin-induced diabetic mice. African Journal of Traditional, Complementary and Alternative Medicines. 2015;**12**(1):90-98

[58] Sabbione AC, Rinaldi G, Añón MC, Scilingo AA. Antithrombotic effects of Amaranthus hypochondriacus proteins in rats. Plant Foods for Human Nutrition. 2016;**71**(1):19-27

[59] Fritz M, Vecchi B, Rinaldi G, Añón MC. Amaranth seed protein hydrolysates have in vivo and in vitro antihypertensive activity. Food Chemistry. 2011;**126**(3):878-884

[60] Zhou XL, Yan BB, Xiao Y, Zhou YM, Liu TY. Tartary buckwheat protein prevented dyslipidemia in high-fat diet-fed mice associated with gut microbiota changes. Food and Chemical Toxicology. 2018;**119**:296-301

[61] Noratto GD, Murphy K, Chew BP. Quinoa intake reduces plasma and liver cholesterol, lessens obesity-associated inflammation, and helps to prevent hepatic steatosis in obese db/db mouse. Food Chemistry. 2019;**287**:107-114

[62] Paśko P, Zagrodzki P, Bartoń H, Chłopicka J, Gorinstein S. Effect of quinoa seeds (Chenopodium quinoa) in diet on some biochemical parameters and essential elements in blood of high fructose-fed rats. Plant Foods for Human Nutrition. 2010;**65**(4):333-338

[63] Foucault AS, Mathé V, Lafont R, Even P, Dioh W, Veillet S, et al. Quinoa extract enriched in 20-hydroxyecdysone protects mice from diet-induced obesity and modulates adipokines expression. Obesity. 2012;**20**(2):270-277

[64] Foucault AS, Even P, Lafont R, Dioh W, Veillet S, Tomé D, et al. Quinoa extract enriched in 20-hydroxyecdysone affects energy homeostasis and intestinal fat absorption in mice fed a high-fat diet. Physiology and Behavior. 2014;**128**:226-231

[65] Ruales J, Grijalva YD, Lopez-Jaramillo P, Nair BM. The nutritional quality of an infant food from quinoa and its effect on the plasma level of insulin-like growth factor-1 (IGF-1) in undernourished children. International Journal of Food Sciences and Nutrition. 2002;**53**(2):143-154

[66] Farinazzi-Machado FMV, Barbalho SM, Oshiiwa M, Goulart R, Pessan Junior O. Use of cereal bars with quinoa (Chenopodium quinoa W.) to reduce risk factors related to cardiovascular diseases. Food Science and Technology. 2012;**32**:239-244

[67] De Carvalho FG, Ovídio PP, Padovan GJ, Jordao Junior AA, Marchini JS, Navarro AM. Metabolic parameters of postmenopausal women after quinoa or corn flakes intake–A prospective and double-blind study. International Journal of Food Sciences and Nutrition. 2014;**65**(3):380-385

[68] Navarro-Perez D, Radcliffe J, Tierney A, Jois M. Quinoa seed lowers serum triglycerides in overweight and obese subjects: A dose-response randomized controlled clinical trial. Current Developments in Nutrition. 2017;**1**(9):e001321

Chapter 6

The Importance of Buckwheat as a Pseudocereal: Content and Stability of Its Main Bioactive Components

Amela Džafić and Sanja Oručević Žuljević

Abstract

The production of various bakery and non-bakery products based on buckwheat with components that positively affect health (fiber, antioxidants, and/or minerals), the optimization of recipes and technological process parameters, as well as giving character to final products in terms of their sensory acceptability and potential functional properties, gained significant interest last few years. Therefore, buckwheat products such as bread, biscuits, snacks, noodles, and cakes are commercialized and increasingly consumed. In addition, the use of non-bakery buckwheat products, such as tea, sprouts, honey, and other products, is becoming more common. In order to obtain potentially functional food with buckwheat of high nutritional quality, it is important to understand the effect of processing on bioactive components. The baking process, inevitable in the production of bakery products, is especially important. It is also important to understand the effect of storage on bioactive components. To this end, in the light of available literature, this chapter will provide an overview of bioactive components in buckwheat and discuss their stability in buckwheat and its products during processing and storage.

Keywords: common and Tartary buckwheat products, sensory acceptability, functional properties, effect of processing and storage, stability of bioactive components

1. Introduction

Buckwheat is an annual herbaceous plant that botanically belongs to the order *Polygonales*, family *Polygonaceae*, genus *Fagopyrum* [1], but in terms of processing, similar use, chemical composition, and the seed structure itself, it is similar to cereals. It is therefore often classified as a pseudocereal [2, 3]. In the genus *Fagopyrum*, 15 species were discovered and described, among which nine have agricultural and nutritional value. However, only two species are most commonly grown: common (*Fagopyrum esculentum* Moench) and Tartary buckwheat (*Fagopyrum Tataricum* L.). Common buckwheat is the most common and cultivated species from temperate Europe to Japan, while Tartary buckwheat is grown in some mountainous areas [4].

Buckwheat grains are the main form of consumption of this pseudocereal. Hulled grains are mostly used for human consumption in the form of breakfast cereals or as flour for the production of various bakery products (bread, cakes, snacks) and noodles enriched with buckwheat flour (0.3–60%), buckwheat-improved non-bakery products (tea, honey, and tarhana) [5] and products made of buckwheat husks such as pillows, quilts, mattresses, collars, eye masks, and children's toys [6]. In addition to flour and groats, buckwheat sprouts are increasingly used to improve bakery products [5, 7].

Since buckwheat is gluten-free, these products can be included in a gluten-free diet for patients with gluten intolerance [8, 9].

The addition of buckwheat into bakery products is of particular importance. This pseudocereal is gaining increasing attention as potentially functional food [4, 10]. Namely, buckwheat is recognized as a good source of nutritious proteins, lipids, dietary fiber and minerals and, in combination with other components that have a positive impact on health such as phenolic components and sterols, it is attracting increasing attention as a functional food. *In vitro* and *in vivo* studies have shown that the consumption of buckwheat and products enriched with this pseudocereal is associated with a wide range of biological and health activities: hypocholesterolemic, hypoglycaemic, anticancer, and anti-inflammatory. According to the recent phytochemical and pharmacological researches polysaccharides of buckwheat present also important bioactive components with numerous biological activities [11].

Buckwheat is the only pseudocereal that contains rutin, which has shown anti-inflammatory, anticancer, antiatherogenic, and antioxidant activity [4, 12]. Buckwheat protein extracts are associated with anticancer and cholesterol-lowering effects in animals [13, 14]. Apparently, the incorporation of buckwheat into bread results in significantly lower blood glucose and insulin responses compared to white wheat bread [15]. Buckwheat grain contains very rare D-*chiro*-inositol, which has been associated with reducing the symptoms of type 2 diabetes mellitus (non-insulin-dependent diabetes mellitus) [16].

2. Bioactive components in buckwheat

2.1 Proteins

Buckwheat proteins have a high biological value thanks to a well-balanced amino acid composition. The protein content of buckwheat is relatively lower than the protein content of legumes. However, the amino acid score of buckwheat protein is 100 and the content of essential amino acids corresponds to the recommended amino acid intake for children and adults [17].

They are rich in lysine, which is the first limiting amino acid of plant proteins, and arginine [18, 19]. However, the content of glutamine and proline is much lower compared to wheat [20], and threonine and methionine are the first and second limiting acids in buckwheat. Furthermore, Giménez-Bastida et al. [5] stated that buckwheat proteins are rich in albumin and globulin and that they are very poor in prolamin and gluten. Therefore, buckwheat flour is suitable for use in the diet of people with celiac disease due to its low non-toxic prolamin content [21]. The protein content in buckwheat flour is significantly higher compared to rice, wheat, corn, millet, and sorghum flour. While it is lower only compared to the protein content of oat flour [19]. Guo et al. [22] pointed out that the average protein content in buckwheat is 12.94%.

The digestibility of buckwheat proteins is about 80%, which is lower compared to proteins of animal origin such as hemoglobin and ovalbumin. However, it is higher than cereal proteins (e.g., sorghum 55–59%; corn 66–75%) and has a value approximate to rice bran (89%) and wheat germ (77–93%). Despite the balanced composition of essential amino acids, the bioavailability of buckwheat protein after digestion is not complete. Relatively low digestibility is attributed to the molecular structure of buckwheat protein and the presence of antinutritive factors in flour and protein isolates [17].

Buckwheat, along with other pseudocereals such as quinoa and amaranth, is recommended for use in creating new value-added bakery products because it can provide high levels of essential amino acids in the human diet [23].

The literature states that buckwheat proteins have many unique physiological functions, such as treating chronic diseases in humans, reducing serum cholesterol, suppressing gallstones and tumors, inhibiting angiotensin I-converting enzyme (ACE), and so on [17, 24, 25]. An ACE inhibitory tripeptide (Gly-Pro-Pro) was isolated and identified from common buckwheat [26]. In humans, buckwheat consumption has also been associated with a lower prevalence of hyperglycemia and improved glucose tolerance in people with diabetes [27]. Since many health benefits of buckwheat are inherently related to peptide radical binding activity from digested proteins, it is hypothesized that buckwheat protein hydrolysis may release peptide fragments capable of stabilizing reactive oxygen kinds and inhibiting lipid oxidation. By in vitro digestion of buckwheat protein six peptide fractions were obtained, whereas LC-MS/MS identified Trp-Pro-Leu, Val-Pro-Trp, and Val-Phe-Pro-Trp (IV), Pro-Trp (V), and tryptophan (VI) as the prominent peptides/amino acid in these fractions [28]. Six peptides DVWY (H-Asp-Val-Trp-Tyr-OH), FDART (H-Phe-Asp-Ala-Arg-Thr-OH), FQ (H-Phe-Gln-OH), VAE (H-Val-Ala-Glu-OH), VVG (H-Val-Val-Gly-OH), and WTFR (H-Trp-Thr-Phe-Arg-OH) identified from buckwheat sprouts fermented with *Lac*tobacillus Plantarum revealed significant blood pressure-lowering effect, thereby the most potent were DVWY, FQ, and VVG [29]. From the seeds of common buckwheat were purified two peptides (Fa-AMP1 and Fa-AMP2) which have antimicrobial properties [30]. Studies have shown that buckwheat protein extracts show anticancer activity, activity of lowering cholesterol, as well as anti-constipation and anti-obesity activities in animals [13, 17, 24]. An unusual antitumor protein TBWSP31 isolated from water-soluble Tartary buckwheat extracts was also examined [31].

2.2 Phenolic components

Many health benefits of buckwheat are attributed to the high content of phenolic components and high antioxidant activity [18]. Whole grain buckwheat was found to contain 2–5 times more phenolic components than barley and oats, while the husk and bran of buckwheat have 2–7 times higher antioxidant activity compared to barley, triticale, and oats [32, 33]. The research by Begić et al. [34] showed that Tartary buckwheat contains about 20 times more total phenol content and that it shows antioxidant activity nine times higher than common buckwheat.

Among the polyphenolic components present in buckwheat, those from the group of flavonoids, and among them rutin, are the most important ones.

2.2.1 Flavonoids

The presence and amount of flavonoids in buckwheat grain make it specific compared to cereals, which contain small amounts of flavonoids. This group of polyphenolic components is the basic antioxidant of buckwheat [35, 36]. Buckwheat is considered to be one of the best dietary sources of rutin [36]. The content and composition of flavonoids are different in different types of buckwheat. In general, the flavonoid content in *F. Tataricum* (40 mg/g) is higher than in *F. esculentum* (10 mg/g), reaching concentrations of 100 mg/g in flowers, leaves, and stems [37]. The content of flavonoids in Tartary buckwheat can be up to 7% [38].

Flavonoids demonstrate a protective effect in lipid oxidation in vitro as "scavengers" of free radicals and metal chelators [39]. They generally occur as O-glycosides in which one or more hydroxyl groups are bound to sugars.

Six flavonoids were isolated and identified from whole buckwheat grains: rutin, quercetin, orientin, isoorientin, vitexin, and isovitexin. The presence of rutin and isovitexin was found in hulled grain while buckwheat husk contained all 6 flavonoids [40, 41]. Buckwheat is the only pseudocereal that contains rutin and is, therefore, a useful source of this flavonoid [25]. Except in buckwheat, rutin has not been detected in cereals and pseudocereals [41, 42]. Rutin (quercetin-3-O-β-rutinoside), a secondary metabolite present in buckwheat, is the best-known glycoside derived from flavonol quercetin. Buckwheat is considered the best source of dietary rutin. Buckwheat grains (groats and husk) and sprouts are important sources of rutin and their content depends on the type and conditions of growth [43, 44]. It is important to develop new well-adaptive varieties with a high content of rutin, and improved biological value of the proteins [45].

Tartary buckwheat groats contain more rutin—80.94 mg/g dry matter (DM) than common buckwheat groats—0.20 mg/g DM [46, 47] while Tartary buckwheat sprouts have 2,2 times more rutin than common buckwheat sprouts [48]. Li et al. [49] stated that Tartary buckwheat can contain up to 100 times more rutin than common buckwheat.

Rutin has attracted much attention mainly because of its many health benefits observed in vitro and in vivo: anti-inflammatory, antidiabetic, hypocholesterolemic, antiatherogenic, antiatherosclerotic, and anticancer ones [4, 12, 36, 50–53] and its activity are related to antioxidant capacity [54]. Furthermore, rutin may be effective in preventing the toxic effects of methotrexate on the kidneys [55].

Rutin has relaxing effects on smooth muscles and is effective in preventing capillary apoplexy and retinal bleeding, lowers high blood pressure and shows antioxidant activity and lipid peroxidation activity. It also has lipid-lowering activity by reducing dietary cholesterol absorption, as well as reducing plasma and liver cholesterol [56, 57]. In addition, possibilities of rutin as a new strategy for the prevention of type 2 diabetes are noted [58]. Alkaline luminol chemiluminescence and electron spin resonance analysis revealed the formation of the rutin-ovalbumin complex which significantly increases the radical-binding activity in rutin. Rutin has also demonstrated antioxidant activity against hydroxyl radicals in a DNA protection test [59].

Quercetin (quercetin-3-ramnoside) is another glycoside present in buckwheat in concentrations ranging from 0.01 to 0.05% DM in Tartary and from 0.54 to 1.80% DM in common buckwheat [46, 60]. Isoquercetin (quercetin-3-glucoside) is present in buckwheat hypocotyl (1.4 μM/g DM) [61] and has been shown to exhibit antidiabetic and anticancer activity [36, 49, 62, 63]. Quercetin, an aglycone of rutin, is present in hulled grain (semolina) of buckwheat (0.001 mg/g DM) and husk (0.009–0.029 mg/g DM) in lower concentrations than rutin [18, 47]. Quercetin is the most studied flavonoid, primarily due to its pronounced antioxidant activity, as well as significant absorption in the digestive tract. It is predominantly in the form of glycoside as rutin (quercetin-3-O-beta-rutinoside). In addition to this, kaempferol-3-O-rutinoside and quercetin 3-O-rutinoside-3'-O-β glucopyranoside have been found in buckwheat seeds [49, 64].

Three flavonoids from Tartary buckwheat bran: quercetin, isoquercetin and rutin were evaluated as R-glucosidase inhibitors (controlling blood glucose) using fluorescence spectroscopy and enzyme kinetics. The R-glucosidase activity was clearly influenced by extractives (mostly rutin) and their hydrolysis products (a mixture of quercetin, isoquercetin, and rutin) from buckwheat bran [65].

Recent research relating to the examination of the antiviral activity of rutin in the treatment of patients with COVID-19 symptoms have been topical [66, 67].

In addition to rutin, catechins, the antioxidant activity of which is higher than the antioxidant activity of rutin, were isolated from ethanol extracts of buckwheat groats. Four catechins were isolated and their structures were determined as: (−)-epicatechin, (+)-catechin-7-O-β-D-glucopyranoside, (−)-epicatechin 3-O-p-hydroxybenzoate, and (−)-epicatechin 3-O-(3,4-di-O-methyl)gallate [68]. The following components from the catechin group were identified in buckwheat: catechin, epicatechin, catechin glucoside (A or B isomers), catechin gallate, epicatechin gallate, epicatechin-O-3,4-dimethylgallate, epiaphzelchin-(4—8)-epicatechin-3,4-O- dimethylgallate, while catechin-3,4-O- dimethylgallate was identified in thermally treated buckwheat and epiaphzelchin- (4—6) -epicatechin was identified in green buckwheat [69].

These ingredients in plant tissue are influenced by numerous environmental factors such as ultraviolet (UV) radiation, harvest time and damage caused by pests, and genetic and aging-related factors. Studies have shown significant positive correlations between the mean altitude of the growth site and the amount of individual phenolic antioxidants [70, 71]. Buckwheat, as a source of rutin, can be successfully grown in Mediterranean conditions, too [72]. Flavon-3-glycosides present in buckwheat (vitexin, isovitexin, orientin, and homoorientin), anthocyanin and proanthocyanin content [61] and the presence of squalene, epicatechin, and vitamin E [73] make buckwheat a good antioxidant source in the human diet.

2.2.2 Phenolic acids

Phenolic acids in buckwheat also contribute to its antioxidant activity. In the grain of different varieties of Tartary buckwheat, p-hydroxybenzoic, ferulic and protocatechuic stand out, and other acids, including p-coumaric, gallic, caffeic, vanillic, and syringic acid, were also detected [74]. Several phenolic acids have been described during the flowering of different varieties of buckwheat: chlorogenic, p-anisic, salicylic, and methoxycinnamic [75].

2.3 Vitamins

Buckwheat is also an important source of vitamins, especially those of the B group. The total content of B vitamins, including B1 (thiamine, 2.2–3.3 μg/g DM), B2 (riboflavin, 10.6 μg/g DM), B3 (niacin, 18 μg/g), B5 (pantothenic acid, 11 μg/g) and B6 (pyridoxine, 1.5 μg/g) is higher in Tartary buckwheat compared to common buckwheat. The levels of vitamin C indicated for it in the literature go as high as 50 μg/g DM while its content, as well as the total amount of vitamins B1 and B6, increases by germination of buckwheat and, consequently, the content of vitamin C in buckwheat sprouts reaches 250 μg/g DM [4, 54, 76, 77]. Vitamin B1 is found in thiamine-binding proteins of buckwheat grains, which, according to Li and Zhang [37] increases the availability of vitamin B1 and improves its stability during storage. The content of vitamin E (tocopherols) in buckwheat is higher compared to wheat, barley, oats, and rye [18]. The most common tocopherol in buckwheat is γ-tocopherol. In addition to γ-tocopherol, α- and δ-tocopherol have also been identified in buckwheat [78]. The concentration of total tocopherols in buckwheat grains ranges from 14.3 to 21.7 mg/kg [79]. Tocopherols, along with the other components mentioned above, make buckwheat a good antioxidant source in the human diet. Tocotrienols were not detected in buckwheat [80, 81], while Piironen et al. [82] identified traces of tocotrienols in whole buckwheat grains. High levels of vitamin E intake are associated with a reduction in cardiovascular disease, a reduction in the risk of Alzheimer's disease, and an improvement in the immune system [73].

2.4 Isoprenoids

Squalene is an isoprenoid component that has six isoprene units and antioxidant activity and is widely produced in buckwheat plants. Squalene protects cells from radicals, strengthens the immune system, and reduces the risk of various types of cancer. There are some differences between buckwheat species, especially in the content of squalene and rutin [73].

2.5 Phagopyritols

Buckwheat grains contain a very rare D-*chiro*-inositol, which is mostly found in the form of phagopyritols [18]. Phagopyritols are mono-, di- and trigalactosyl derivatives of D- *chiro*-inositol and are called phagopyritol B1, B2, and B3. Phagopyritols A1, A2, and A3 have been identified as isomers of phagopyritols B1, B2, and B3 [83–85]. Phagopyritols are concentrated in aleurone and embryonic grain cells, with phagopyritol B1 (0.392 mg/g DM of integral common buckwheat semolina) being the most abundant. D-*chiro*-inositol, free form, is present in lower concentrations (0.21–0.42 mg/g DM) [18].

So far, several studies have described the role of D-*chiro*-inositol and phagopyritol as molecules that exhibit insulin-like activity [18, 86, 87]. In particular, D-*chiro*-inositol has attracted much interest due to its ability to lower glucose in animal models [88], and an important number of studies have shown that chemically synthesized D-*chiro*-inositol lowers elevated plasma glucose levels [89, 90]. Although no studies have been conducted to date to explore the effects of D-*chiro*-inositol and phagopyritol in humans, these components may have positive effects in the treatment of diabetes. In animal models, D-*chiro*-inositol has been associated with a reduction in the symptoms of type 2 diabetes mellitus [16]. The potential of D-*chiro*-inositol in the treatment of polycystic ovary syndrome has been extensively investigated [57, 91–93].

2.6 Phytosterols

Buckwheat is also significant for its phytosterol content. Phytosterols present in buckwheat, although in low concentrations, also show a positive effect in lowering blood cholesterol levels. In addition, phytosterol intake significantly reduces in vivo cholesterol absorption. Buckwheat phytosterols are present throughout the grain, but their content varies by grain parts [37]. The most abundant phytosterol in buckwheat flour is β-sitosterol (0.86 mg/g DM) and makes up about 70% of total sterols, followed by campesterol (0.11 mg/g DM) and stigmasterol (0.02 mg/g DM) [94].

According to the research of Dziedzic et al. [95]. the sterols content in Tartary buckwheat whole grains was 15,398 mg/kg of lipids and the most prevalent was the β-sitosterol (10,944 mg/kg of lipids).

2.7 Iminosugars

D-fagomin is a minor component from the group of iminosugars detected in the dehulled grain of common buckwheat which shows a glucose-lowering effect [96, 97].

Similar to D-fagomin, other imino sugars such as 1-deoxynojirimycin (DNJ) are intestinal glucosidase inhibitors, associated with a reduced risk of developing insulin resistance, gaining weight, and suffering from excess potentially pathogenic bacteria [97, 98]. Anthraquinone emodin is present in buckwheat concentrations between 1.72 and 2.71 mg/kg DM [99]. Due to the wide range of biological activities that emodin exhibits, it can be considered an important bioactive factor in buckwheat [100].

2.8 Other components

Along with vitamins, other components were detected, such as glutathione (1.10 mmol/g DM in buckwheat groats), phytic acid (35–38 mg/g DM in bran), carotenoids (2.10 mg/g DM in grain), and melatonin (470 pg/g DM in groats). These components may contribute to the antioxidant activity of buckwheat [4, 47].

Both types of buckwheat, common and Tartary, have a high tannin content (1.76 and 1.54%). Tannins isolated from buckwheat showed a relatively high level of activity against *Listeria monocytogenes* [101].

It has also been found that γ-aminobutyric acid (GABA) and 2″-hydroxynicotianamine (2HN) serve as functional components in buckwheat. Grains and sprouts contain GABA, while 2HN was identified in flour. Literature states that these components lower blood pressure in humans and inhibit the activity of angiotensin I-converting enzyme (ACE) [102–104]. Suzuki et al. [105] quantified GABA and 2HN concentrations in common and Tartary buckwheat leaves 14, 28, and 42 days after sowing (DAS). The concentration of GABA reached a peak at 42 DAS, while the concentration of 2HN decreased with the age of the plant.

3. Stability of bioactive components in buckwheat and its products during processing

It is well known that processing can cause chemical changes in food products. Therefore, it is important to consider the effects on bioactive components in buckwheat. Today, there are several technological processes related to buckwheat, which will be presented below.

3.1 Milling

Milling is one of the technological processes that is inevitable during the processing of buckwheat into flour. During the processing of buckwheat grains into white flour, the husk and outer layers are separated, which lowers the ratio of fibers, minerals, and polyphenolic components.

Hung and Morita [106] explored the possibility of improving the functionality of buckwheat flour by successively milling buckwheat and they found that in 16 different fractions of flour the content of ferulic acid and rutin increases with an increased ratio of outer grain layers. The same authors found that the antiradical activity on DPPH extracts of free and bound polyphenolic components of buckwheat, the fraction of the successive milling of buckwheat is highest for fractions containing external grain parts. Additionally, better antiradical activity on DPPH was registered for extracts of free polyphenolic components compared to extracts of bound polyphenolic components in buckwheat grain.

Inglett et al. [107] examined the antioxidant activity of ethanolic extracts of four types of commercial buckwheat flour and found the highest antiradical activity on DPPH in buckwheat flour containing a high ratio of husk and aleurone layer, while the lowest antiradical activity was registered in white flour consisting exclusively of the endosperm. The highest content of total polyphenolic components and total flavonoids was registered in whole buckwheat flour. Gallardo et al. [108] established that the content of rutin in buckwheat flour is 0.7 mg/100 g and 11.2 mg/100 g in buckwheat husk.

A recent study found that the buckwheat protein contents decreased from the exterior to the interior parts of the groats [109]. Significantly higher content of amino acids, fatty acids, polyphenols, and flavonoids was found in the bran of Tartary buckwheat, compared to the flour [110].

It should be noted that the milling conditions should be adapted to the type of buckwheat. The granulation composition of common and Tartary buckwheat flour differed under the same milling conditions and affected the physical characteristics of the obtained flour fractions. Tartary buckwheat flour contained larger fractions compared to common buckwheat flour under the same milling conditions [111]. By adjusting the grinding and knowing the content of different components in the fractions of Tartary buckwheat, it is possible to obtain products of different nutritional value [45, 111].

3.2 Heat treatment

The number of studies researching the effects of heat treatment on buckwheat foods has increased significantly. Today, many new thermal techniques are used in the food industry to improve the quality of functional buckwheat food. The extrusion process has become important in the production of pasta, ready-to-eat cereals, snacks, animal feeds, and textured plant proteins. Microwave heating has gained popularity in food processing due to the ability of this technique to achieve high heating rates, significantly reduce cooking time, provide more uniform heating and safe handling. This technique could change the taste and nutritional properties of food to a lesser extent, as opposed to conventional heating during the cooking process [112]. However, data on the effects of heat treatments on the antioxidant capacity of buckwheat and its products are still limited. In general, most studies are aimed at determining the effect of heat treatment on the content of total phenols and flavonoids due to their role in the management of human health and diseases.

It was established that the heat treatment of buckwheat causes changes in its chemical composition and, above all, that it affects the functional properties of the selected bioactive components. The results published so far on the effects of the heat treatment on buckwheat grain and processed flour are contradictory.

One of the first studies was conducted by Dietrych-Szostak and Oleszek [40] who examined the effect of heat processing on flavonoid content in hulled grains and buckwheat husks by removing the husk using heat. Removing the husk from buckwheat grain by applying heat treatment resulted in a product that was both visually and chemically different. The peeling process removed primarily the multitude of tannins and crude fibers that are naturally present in the husk. As for the concentration of total flavonoids, dehulling process with different temperature treatments caused a drastic reduction of the total flavonoid concentration in the grain (by 75% of the control) and smaller but significant (15–20%) reduction in the hulls.

Kreft et al. [12] compared the content of rutin in buckwheat products with its content in the raw materials used to obtain these products. Noodles prepared with 70% of integral buckwheat flour contained much less rutin (78 mg/kg DM) compared to the integral buckwheat flour (218 mg/kg DM) out of which they were produced. As a possible explanation for this reduction in rutin content in the product, the authors cited the presence and activity of an enzyme that degrades rutin, flavonol 3-glucosidase, during dough mixing. The presence of this enzyme in buckwheat was confirmed by Suzuki et al. [113]. In raw (uncooked) hulled buckwheat grain (raw buckwheat semolina) the rutin content was 230 mg/kg DM, while in pre-cooked hulled buckwheat grain its content was 88 mg/kg DM. The aforementioned authors explained the established reduction of rutin content in hulled buckwheat grain due to hydrothermal treatment by possible degradation of rutin molecules or its combination with some other molecules, in such a way that it becomes insoluble in the applied solvent. A similar reduction in rutin content was observed during bread production in different combinations of wheat and Tartary buckwheat flour (100:0; 70:30; 50:50; and 0:100) where the effect of making bread and baking on the content of rutin, quercetin, and polyphenols and the antioxidant activity of said loaves was examined. After baking, rutin (0.47 mg/g) was present in bread which is made of 100% Tartary buckwheat flour, together with quercetin (4.83 mg/g). The dough that this bread was made of contained a lower concentration of rutin and greater concentration of quercetin compared to flour used to prepare it; wherein 0.0175 mmol of rutin degraded with the addition of water and yeast to Tartary buckwheat flour, and 0.0149 mmol of quercetin was obtained at the same time. This indicates that 85% of the rutin was converted to quercetin by adding water and yeast to the flour [114].

Degradation of rutin can be the result of activities of the rutin-degrading enzyme found in buckwheat. This enzyme is stable and active at pH 5–7 and below 40°C. Based on the comparison of the level of concentration, it appears that quercetin is more stable compared to rutin in the process of proofing and baking bread. There were no significant differences in the content of rutin and quercetin between the bread crumb and crust. Additionally, the results showed a reduction in the total polyphenol content in all samples of bread as a result of the heat treatment in the baking process [112].

The obtained results were consistent with the results of the authors Alvarez-Jubete et al. [21] which showed a significant decrease in the concentration of total polyphenols, particularly phenolic acids in bread made of common buckwheat flour (0.65 mg GAE/g) compared to the concentrations of these components in buckwheat grain (3.23 mg GAE/g). During the process of mixing and proofing the bread, there was a modest increase in the concentration of total polyphenols in bread samples made with 100% wheat flour and 100% Tartary buckwheat flour, and a slight reduction in the other samples, containing a combination of both kinds of flour (70:30 and 50:50).

Reductions in polyphenol content and antioxidant activity were also reported during baking of bread samples prepared in different combinations (90:10; 80:20; and 70:30) of rice and buckwheat flour (wholemeal and white) relative to their content in flours. It was noticed that the baking process resulted in a higher percentage of reduction in total polyphenols in bread samples made white buckwheat flour, while only minor or insignificant changes were observed in lower percentages (10 and 20%) in samples with wholemeal buckwheat flour, and only the sample with 30% of wholemeal buckwheat flour had a decrease of about 17%. In addition, the decrease in antioxidant activity was more pronounced in bread samples prepared with white buckwheat flour. During baking, there was a loss in rutin content in bread samples relative to its assumed (calculated) content, and this loss increased with increasing the proportion of buckwheat flour, both types (wholemeal and white), in the range of 4.57–40.4%. The opposite trend was observed in the quercetin content, which increased from 1.5 to 7 times, probably due to the hydrolysis of rutin into quercetin [115].

Similar results were shown in bread samples produced with the addition of buckwheat in the amount of 15 g/100 g and 30 g/100 g. A decrease in the content of total phenols, total flavonoids, and antioxidant activity in bread samples relative to their content in flour was found. The content of total flavonoids in bread samples was 2 to 4 times lower compared to its content in flour [116].

The thermal treatment of Tartary buckwheat bran and flour significantly reduced the content of fatty acids, polysaccharides, and polyphenols. As for the content of amino acids and total flavonoids, their content in bran after heat treatment decreased, while increased in the flour of Tartary buckwheat [110].

In addition to bread and cakes, a decrease in the content of bioactive components was observed in the production and cooking of other products with the addition of buckwheat such as spaghetti, pasta, noodles, etc. A decrease in the content of free (about 74.5%) and bound (about 80%) phenolic components "farm to table", i.e., from flour to cooked spaghetti with buckwheat was found. Regarding the content of total phenolic components, the spaghetti production process (mixing, extrusion, and drying) caused a loss of 45.9%, which the authors explain by the increase in temperature during the extrusion process and the high temperature (about 95°C) reached during drying. Further degradation of phenolic components was found after cooking spaghetti. The boiling process caused the degradation of 52.9% of the total phenolic components. This degradation was significantly different ($p < 0.05$) compared to post-production degradation. This effect can be attributed to the solubility of phenolic components in boiled water. Of the total phenolic components that were present in the spaghetti after the drying process, 11.6% were dissolved in water after cooking [117].

Biney and Beta [118] also reported that the production and cooking process led to a reduction in phenol content and antioxidant activity in spaghetti enriched with buckwheat flour and bran. The production process did not cause statistically ($p < 0.05$) significant changes in the content of total phenols between flour mixtures and uncooked products. However, cooking significantly reduced total phenols in all spaghetti samples. Although the addition of buckwheat flour resulted in a significantly higher content of these components in all spaghetti samples, the average percentage of decrease in total cooking phenols due to cooking was higher in samples containing buckwheat flour or bran, compared to control samples prepared from semolina. The production and cooking process also led to a significant reduction in the content of rutin and total flavonoids in spaghetti samples. The higher the proportion of buckwheat in the spaghetti formulation, the greater the losses in rutin content.

The results of similar research (pasta enriched with buckwheat flour in the amount of 20%) showed a reduction of about 44% of total phenolic components after cooking compared to their content in pasta after drying; 8.37% of total phenols from dried pasta was present in the water in which it was boiled, and 35.63% was degraded. The cooking process reduced the rutin content by about 8.50%. During cooking, rutin was converted from its bound form to quercetin, which is shown in the increase of quercetin content by about 20%. The results also showed that catechin showed a minimum tolerance to the cooking process, with a loss of about 57% [119].

Furthermore, the autoclaving of buckwheat grains caused a decrease in free and an increase in bound phenolic forms in flour. Similarly, this was found in noodles produced by adding this flour to the formulation with wheat flour, compared to the content of these components in noodles produced in the same way with flour obtained from untreated buckwheat grains. Although autoclaving caused an initial reduction in rutin in treated grain flours, it prevented further degradation and conversion of rutin to quercetin in uncooked and cooked samples obtained from these flours, causing a possible improvement in the sensory acceptability of noodles. The loss of phenolic components in noodle samples with added buckwheat flour during cooking (48.1–61.1%) was at the same level as in the control sample with wheat flour only, indicating that buckwheat-containing pasta can maintain the quality during cooking [120].

Cho and Lee [121] examined the thermal stability of rutin in wheat instant fried noodles fortified with rutin-enriched material (REM) from buckwheat milling fractions. The noodles were fried at different temperatures (150, 170, and 190°C) during different periods of time (1, 2, and 3 minutes). Also, noodles were placed in boiling water at different periods (0, 3, and 6 minutes) to examine the effect of cooking on rutin content. The results showed that different temperatures and frying times did not negatively affect the rutin content, while a marked loss of rutin was observed after cooking the noodles.

However, the results of another study showed a reduction in bioactive components in buckwheat products during various heat treatment processes and reported an increase in the total antioxidant activity in buckwheat sprouts and shoots after autoclaving treatment. Furthermore, an increase of 20% and a reduction of 7% of total phenols were observed in buckwheat sprouts and shoot respectively [122].

Contradictory results were also found by Zieliński et al. [123] during extrusion of buckwheat, which showed a decrease in antioxidant capacity accompanied by a reduction in rutin and isovitexin, but at the same time an increase in free phenolic acids and those freed from ester bonds. The authors stated that the reported increase in phenolic acids could be due to the increased release of these bioactive components from the matrix, making them available for extraction. The same authors report that, although the extrusion caused a marked reduction in antioxidant content in hulled buckwheat grain, the amount of bioactive component in hulled buckwheat grain after thermal treatment was still significant, resulting in a decrease in antioxidant activity of only 10%.

Hes et al. [124] also reported contradictory results when testing the impact of cooking in water on the antioxidant properties and dietary fiber of hulled buckwheat grain. It was shown that cooking in water for 30 minutes in a ratio of 2:1 (water: grain) has no negative effects on the nutritional characteristics of the hulled buckwheat grain. Extracts of cooked hulled grain showed a significantly higher content of polyphenols and total dietary fiber compared to raw grain. The detected higher content of polyphenols in cooked hulled grain is explained by the authors as a result of their partial release from the bound form of the protein as a result of cooking. Additionally, phenols can also be associated with other components such as carbohydrates. In terms of individual phenolic components, a significantly higher content of catechin particularly stands out, and, in contrast to that, a considerably lower content of p-coumaric acid in the extracts of cooked buckwheat grain compared to the extracts of the raw buckwheat grain. Cooking did not cause any changes in rutin content.

It has been recognized that the possible beneficial effects of phytochemicals present in buckwheat may be related to the inherent antioxidant capacity of these components. Therefore, during the last decade, the relationship between antioxidant capacity and these components after heat treatment has been exposed. The antioxidant capacity of buckwheat products is linked to flavonoid concentrations after hydrothermal treatment [125]. Kreft et al. [12] described significant correlations between rutin content and antioxidant activity of buckwheat grain and buckwheat food products. Chlopicka et al. [116] found positive and significant correlations between total phenols and antioxidant activity in buckwheat bread samples, as well as between total phenols and antioxidant activity of buckwheat bread samples, and, finally, between antioxidant activities themselves. Zhang et al. [126] reported that the baking, heating under steam pressure, and microwave heating of integral buckwheat flour had a statistically significant ($P < 0.05$) effect on the decrease in total flavonoids and antioxidant activity of flour, while the decrease in total phenols in buckwheat flour was less pronounced for all three applied treatments. As a possible explanation, the authors cited the creation of Maillard reaction products, which react with Folin-Ciocalteu reagent, resulting in masking the actual decrease in polyphenol content.

Similar conclusions regarding the formation of Maillard reaction products were reached by the authors Constantini et al. [127] during the production of bread with the addition of Tartary buckwheat flour, where a loss in the total antioxidant capacity and content of total polyphenols and flavonoids was observed, relative to their values in flour mixtures. The aforementioned authors pointed out that it is possible that the real reduction is greater than what was found in this study. As an explanation, they stated that heat treatment of cereals and pseudocereals, such as during baking, can also result in the synthesis of substances with antioxidant properties, including certain products of the Maillard reaction that occur in the crust of bread. These syntheses can mask the actual decrease in the content of total phenols and flavonoids (which are able to react with Folin-Ciocalteu reagent), as well as any loss in total antioxidant capacity.

Aside from phenols, other components, such as proteins, appear to be involved in the formation of the antioxidant activity of buckwheat products. The frying hulled buckwheat grain, in addition to reducing antioxidant activity, also resulted in a decrease in protein content and quality, while heat treatment did not show an effect on whole grain proteins [125]. In addition, during thermal treatment, Maillard components are generated due to a chemical reaction between the free amino groups of lysine and the carbonyl groups of reducing sugars [128]. It was observed the formation of Maillard products was caused by heat treatment of both whole and hulled buckwheat grains. Although Maillard components may be harmful to health, they may contribute to an increase in antioxidant activity, masking the actual decrease in total phenolic components, as highlighted in the above studies [125–127]. In addition, it has been suggested that antioxidant capacity may increase as a result of dissociation (separation) of phenolic forms and release of phenols bound to cell walls due to heat treatment followed by polymerization/oxidation of phenolic constituents or by-product generation [122].

The influence of baking on the content of tocopherols in buckwheat bread was investigated. Vitamin E loss was found to be about 30%. Smaller losses were observed in bread samples of 100% buckwheat flour compared to samples in which the share of buckwheat flour was 50% [81]. A significant reduction in vitamin E content (about 63%) in buckwheat was also found during the extrusion process [123].

The importance of common and Tartary buckwheat is generally recognized. However, one should also keep in mind some disadvantages of their application in the bakery in terms of sensory impression. This primarily refers to the particle size and the proportion of bran that can negatively affect the rheological properties of the dough and result in an inappropriate texture of bakery products. In addition, the finished products with Tatary buckwheat may appear a slightly bitter taste [6].

Based on all of the above, it is indicative that the contradictory results obtained so far greatly emphasize the importance of determining the exact composition and ratio of bioactive components. In addition, more studies are needed to identify the effect of heat treatment on the functional components, including proteins and phenolic components, of buckwheat products, in order to ultimately obtain buckwheat of consumption quality. Therefore, processing conditions, such as time and temperature, need to be optimized to preserve the functionality of bioactive components.

3.3 High pressure

High pressure has been shown to be a viable alternative to heat treatment, with no adverse effects such as forming an off flavor, loss of vitamins and phytochemical properties, and discoloration [129]. The effect of high hydrostatic pressure treatment (200 MPa at 2, 4, and 9 minutes) on total antioxidant capacity (TAC), reducing capacity (RC), and rutin content of raw and roasted buckwheat groats were examined. After high-pressure treatment, the content of TAC and rutin differed in the case of raw and fried semolina. The TAC of raw and fried semolina subjected to high-pressure treatment was 16–20% and 12.5–17% lower, respectively, compared to the TAC of untreated semolina. Hydrophilic antioxidants were the main components contributing to the TAC of raw and fried semolina subjected to high-pressure treatment. RC decreased in the case of raw buckwheat (raw semolina), while the rutin content dropped in a shorter time compared to fried semolina. In contrast, overpressure in fried semolina increased the RC formed by hydrophilic antioxidants by 18% when measured by cyclic voltammetry on average and decreased the concentration of rutin after treatment [130].

The results of Zhou et al. [131] suggested that treatment under high pressure at 45 °C improves the nutritional properties of buckwheat compared to untreated and treated under high pressure at room temperature.

3.4 Ionization and radiation

Radiation is a method of treating food to make it safer to eat and to extend its shelf life. Traditionally, this process is used to control surface microorganisms on vegetables and fruits without affecting nutritional quality. Hayashi et al. [132] reduced the microbial load to a lower level by exposing buckwheat grains to soft-electrons without affecting their quality. Chun and Song [133] conducted a study in which aqueous chlorine dioxide, fumaric acid, modified packaging atmosphere enriched with CO_2, and ultraviolet radiation (UV) were combined in the treatment of buckwheat sprouts to improve microbiological quality. A decrease in total aerobic bacteria, yeasts and moulds, and enterobacteria to low levels was observed without affecting sensory quality. However, after the treatment, there was an increase in the concentration of rutin. A comparative study by Orsák et al. [134] studied the effects of UV, microwave, and γ-radiation on three buckwheat samples. Different effects were observed depending on the radiation system and the applied dose on the content of polyphenols and rutin. In addition, it has been described that the content of rutin and flavone C-glycosides is improved in sprouts after exposure to LED (light-emitting diodes) [135].

Therefore, radiation could be offered as a way to increase the half-life of food, maintain sensory quality, improve microbiological quality and increase nutritional value due to bioactive components in buckwheat products. Although public knowledge about radiation remains limited, interest in buying "safe—radiation-enhanced food" is increasing, especially after obtaining information about the potential benefits and risks.

4. Stability of bioactive components in buckwheat and its products during storage

A detailed review of the literature showed that the data on the stability of the most important bioactive components in all types of buckwheat products (bakery and others) during storage is quite limited. Unlike stability during processing, which can still be stated to have been the subject of a significant number of studies in recent years, and that the number of studies is constantly increasing, stability during storage is still almost unexplored. One of the studies that could be related to a certain extent to the mentioned topic is the one conducted by the authors Cho and Lee [121].

Namely, these authors established experimental extraction procedures for preparing rutin-enriched material (REM) from buckwheat milling fractions. Then the REM was used for the fortification of wheat instant fried noodles with rutin. After frying, the noodle samples were stored for 14 days at 60°C and its peroxide value was measured every other day in order to examine the effect of REM on the oxidative stability of the noodles. The monitoring showed that the peroxide number of noodle samples tended to increase with increasing storage time. However, it was noted that the rate of increase in peroxide value was markedly lower in noodle samples with incorporated REM compared to the control sample which did not contain REM. This indicates that the oxidizing improvement of instant fried noodles in storage was reduced using REM. These results can be expected from the high level of rutin in REM, since rutin has strong antioxidant activity [32].

Tabaković et al. [136] found that the most suitable way to store buckwheat seeds for a long period is paper material in order to retain their physiological and morphological properties to the greatest extent.

5. Conclusion

Buckwheat, a pseudocereal belonging to the *Polygonaceae* family, is used as an important raw material for the development of functional foods due to its functionality and content of components such as proteins, flavonoids, phytosterols, phagopyritols, phenolic acids, vitamins, and others. Scientific research confirms many biological and health properties of buckwheat: hypocholesterolemic, hypoglycaemic, anticancer, and anti-inflammatory activity. The increase in the amount of data focused on the positive nutritional and functional characteristics of buckwheat, which affect the prevention and treatment of chronic diseases, reduction of plasma and liver cholesterol, etc., results in an increase in the number of newly created buckwheat-based food products and their increased use in the population's diet. In the category of bakery products, the following ones stand out: buckwheat-enhanced bread, wheat bread enhanced with fermented buckwheat sourdough, buckwheat biscuits and snacks, and many others. However, in order for these products to be of high nutritional quality, it is important to understand the effect of processing on bioactive components. And it is also important to know the effect of storage on bioactive components.

When it comes to processing, there are several processes associated with buckwheat, the first and inevitable one being the milling process. Milling is the processing (conversion) of buckwheat grains into flour, the primary raw material for the production of bakery products. During the processing of buckwheat grains into white flour, the husk and outer layers are separated, which removes the ratio of fibers, minerals, and polyphenolic components. Then there is the process of heat treatment, and baking, which belongs to the category of heat treatment, is also inevitable during the production of bakery products. In general, when it comes to the effects of heat treatment on bioactive components in buckwheat, a considerable amount of research has been conducted so far. However, the results of the conducted studies are contradictory. Although in most cases heat treatment resulted in a decrease in bioactive components, on the other hand, there are studies in which heat treatment did not have a significant effect on bioactive components. Therefore, it is necessary to conduct more studies with an emphasis on optimizing the conditions of heat treatment in order to ultimately obtain buckwheat and buckwheat-based products of appropriate quality for use. Recently, high-pressure treatments and the application of radiation are becoming increasingly important. However, although knowledge about radiation remains limited, there is an increased interest in buying "safe—radiation-enhanced food", especially after obtaining information about the potential benefits and risks.

Although a considerable number of studies have been conducted on the effects of processing, and primarily on the effects of heat treatment, there are still significant gaps in this area. They are primarily related to the fact that most of the conducted studies are aimed at determining the effects of processing on the content of phenolic components, especially flavonoids, due to their recognized role in health benefits. Therefore more research that focuses on the effects of processing on all other bioactive components in buckwheat is needed in the future.

When it comes to the effects of storage, this topic is still almost unexplored. A review of the literature revealed that there is a small number of studies dealing with this topic, and therefore further research is needed to identify the effect of storage on bioactive components of buckwheat products, and ultimately to preserve their quality for as long as possible.

Author details

Amela Džafić* and Sanja Oručević Žuljević
Faculty of Agriculture and Food Sciences, University of Sarajevo, Sarajevo, Bosnia and Herzegovina

*Address all correspondence to: amela.b.dzafic@gmail.com

References

[1] Subhash B, Yadav GS, Singh R, Avasthem RK, Das A, Mohapatra KP, et al. Production technology and multifarious uses of Buckwheat (*Fagopyrum* spp.): A review. Indian Journal of Agronomy. 2018;**63**(4):118-130

[2] Campbell CG. Buckwheat. *Fagopyrum esculentum* Moench. Promoting the conservation and use of underutilized and neglected crops. 19. In: Institute of Plant Genetics and Crop Plant Research, Gatersleben/International Plant Genetic Resources Institute. Rome, Italy: CAB International; 1997

[3] Keskitalo M, Ketoja E, Kontturi M, Maarit M, Pihlava JM, Rantamäki P, et al. Buckwheat—An old crop with new health prospects. NJF Report, Nordic Association of Agricultural Scientists. 2007;**3**(1):23-26

[4] Zhang Z, Zhou M, Tang Y, Li F, Tang Y, Shao J, et al. Bioactive components in functional buckwheat food. Food Research International. 2012;**49**(1):389-395. DOI: 10.1016/j.foodres.2012.07.035

[5] Giménez-Bastida J, Piskula M, Zieliński H. Recent advances in processing and development of buckwheat derived bakery and nonbakery products—A review. Polish Journal of Food and Nutrition Sciences. 2015;**65**(1):9-20. DOI: 10.1515/pjfns-2015-0005

[6] Oručević Žuljević S, Gadžo D. Proizvodnja i prerada heljde u Bosni i Hercegovini—Dosadašnja iskustva i budući izazovi. In: Raspor P, Smole Možina S, editors. Hrana in prehrana za zdravlje, Ajda od njive do zdravlja. Izola. Slovenija: Inštitut za ževila, prehrano in zdravje; 2015. pp. 153-163

[7] Sturza A, Paucean A, Chis MS, Mures V, Vodnar DC, Man SM, et al. Influence of buckwheat and buckwheat sprouts flours on the nutritional and textural parameters of wheat buns. Applied Sciences. 2020;**10**(22):7969-7969. DOI: 10.3390/app10227969

[8] Saturni L, Ferrett G, Bacchetti T. The gluten-free diet: Safety and nutritional quality. Nutrients. 2010;**2**(1):16-34. DOI: 10.3390/nu20100016

[9] Oručević Žuljević S, Akagić A. Flour-based confectionery as functional food. In: Arshad MS, Ahmad MH, editors. Functional Foods—Phytochemicals and Health Promoting Potential. Rijeka: IntechOpen; 2021. DOI: 10.5772/intechopen.95876

[10] Yilmaz HO, Ayhan NY, Meric CS. Buckwheat: A Useful Food and its Effects on Human Health. Current Nutrition and Food Science. 2020;**16**:29-34. DOI: 10.2174/1573401314666180910140021

[11] Ji X, Han L, Liu F, Yin S, Peng Q, Wang M. A mini-review of isolation, chemical properties and bioactivities of polysaccharides from buckwheat (*Fagopyrum* Mill). International Journal of Biological Macromolecules. 2019;**127**:204-209. DOI: 10.1016/j.ijbiomac.2019.01.043

[12] Kreft I, Fabjan N, Yasumoto K. Rutin content in buckwheat (*Fagopyrum esculentum* Moench) food materials and products. Food Chemistry. 2006;**98**(3):508-512. DOI: 10.1016/j.foodchem.2005.05.081

[13] Liu Z, Ishikawa W, Huang X, Tomotake H, Kayashita J, Watanabe H, et al. A buckwheat protein product

suppresses 1,2-dimethylhydrazine-induced colon carcinogenesis in rats by reducing cell proliferation. The Journal of Nutrition. 2001;**131**(6):1850-1853. DOI: 10.1093/jn/131.6.1850

[14] Tomotake H, Yamamoto N, Yanaka N, Ohinata H, Yamazaki R, Kayashita J. High protein buckwheat flour suppresses hypercholesterolemia in rats and gallstone formation in mice by hypercholesterolemic diet and body fat in rats because of its low protein digestibility. Nutrition. 2006;**22**(2):166-173. DOI: 10.1016/j.nut.2005.01.012

[15] Skrabanja V, Liljeberg Elmstahl HG, Kreft I, Björck IM. Nutritional properties of starch in buckwheat products: Studies in vitroand in vivo. Journal of Agricultural and Food Chemistry. 2001;**49**(1):490-496. DOI: 10.1021/jf000779w

[16] Kawa JM, Taylor CG, Przybylski R. Buckwheat concentrate reduces serum glucose in streptozotocin-diabetic rats. Journal of Agricultural and Food Chemistry. 2003;**51**(25):7287-7291. DOI: 10.1021/jf0302153

[17] Jin J, Ikenna C, Ohanenye and Chibuike C, Udenigwe. Buckwheat proteins: Functionality, safety, bioactivity, and prospects as alternative plant-based proteins in the food industry. Critical Reviews in Food Science and Nutrition. 16 Nov 2020:1-13. DOI: 10.1080/10408398.2020.1847027

[18] Wijngaard HH, Arendt EK. Buckwheat—Review. Cereal Chemistry. 2006;**83**(4):391-401. DOI: 10.1094/CC-83-0391

[19] Ahmed A, Khalid N, Ahmad A, Abbasi NA, Latif MSZ, Randhawa MA. Phytochemicals and biofunctional properties of buckwheat. The Journal of Agricultural Science. 2014;**152**:349-369. DOI: 10.1017/S0021859613000166

[20] Aubrecht E, Biac P. Characterization of buckwheat grain proteins and its products. Acta Alimentaria. 2001;**30**:71-80

[21] Alvarez-Jubete L, Arendt EK, Gallagher E. Nutritive value and chemical composition of pseudocereals as gluten-free ingredients. International Journal of Food Sciences and Nutrition. 2009;**60**(Suppl 4):240-257. DOI: 10.1080/09637480902950597

[22] Guo YZ, Chen QF, Yang LY, Huang YH. Analyses of the seed protein contents on the cultivated and wild buckwheat *Fagopyrum esculentum* resources. Genetic Resources and Crop Evolution. 2007;**54**:1465-1472. DOI: 10.1007/s10722-006-9135-z

[23] Škrobot D, Milovanović I, Jovanov P, Pestorić M, Tomić J, Mandić A. Buckwheat, quinoa and amaranth: Good alternatives to nutritious food. Journal on Processing and Energy in Agriculture. 2019;**23**(3):113-116

[24] Tomotake H, Shimaoka I, Kayashita J, Yokoyama F, Nakajoh M, Kato N. A Buckwheat protein product suppresses gallstone formation and plasma cholesterol more strongly than soy protein isolate in hamsters. The Journal of Nutrition. 2000;**130**(7):1670-1674. DOI: 10.1093/jn/130.7.1670

[25] Koyama M, Nakamura C, Nakamura K. Changes in phenols contents from buckwheat sprouts during growth stage. Journal of Food Science and Technology. 2011;**50**(1):86-93. DOI: 10.1007/s13197-011-0316-1

[26] Ma MS, Bae IY, Lee HG, Yang CB. Purification and identification of angiotensin I-converting enzyme

inhibitory peptide from buckwheat (*Fagopyrum esculentum* Moench). Food Chemistry. 2006;**96**(1):36-42. DOI: 10.1016/j.foodchem.2005.01.052

[27] Zhang HW, Zhang YH, Lu MJ, Tong WJ, Cao GW. Comparison of hypertension, dyslipidaemia and hyperglycaemia between buckwheat seed-consuming and non-consuming Mongolian-Chinese populations in Inner Mongolia, China. Clinical and Experimental Pharmacology and Physiology. 2007;**34**(9):838-844. DOI: 10.1111/j.1440-1681.2007

[28] Ma Y, Xiong YL, Zhai JJ, Zhu HN, Dziubla T. Fractionation and evaluation of radical scavenging peptides from in vitro digests of buckwheat protein. Food Chemistry. 2010;**118**(3):582-588. DOI: 10.1016/j.foodchem.2009.05.024

[29] Koyama MK, Naramoto T, Nakajima T, Aoyama T, Watanabe M, Nakamura K. Purification and identification of antihypertensive peptides from fermented buckwheat sprouts. Journal of Agricultural and Food Chemistry. 2013;**61**(12):3013-3021. DOI: 10.1021/jf305157y

[30] Fujimura M, Minami Y, Watanabe K, Tadera K. Purification, characterization, and sequencing of a novel type of antimicrobial peptides, Fa-AMP1 and Fa-AMP2, from seeds of buckwheat (*Fagopyrum esculentum* Moench.). Bioscience, Biotechnology, and Biochemistry. 2003;**67**(8):1636-1642. DOI: 10.1271/bbb.67.1636

[31] Guo XN, Zhu KX, Zhang H, Yao HY. Anti-tumor activity of a novel protein obtained from tartary buckwheat. International Journal of Molecular Sciences. 2010;**11**(12):5201-5211. DOI: 10.3390/ijms11125201

[32] Holasova M, Fiedlerova V, Smrcinova H, Orsak M, Lachman J, Vavreinova S. Buckwheat—The source of antioxidant activity in functional foods. Food Research International. 2002;**35**(1-2):207-211. DOI: 10.1016/S0963-9969(01)00185-5

[33] Zdunczyk Z, Flis M, Zieliński H, Wroblewska M, Antoszkiewicz Z, Juskiewicz J. In vitro antioxidant activities of barley, husked oat, naked oat, triticale, and buckwheat wastes and their influence on the growth and biomarkers of antioxidant status in rats. Journal of Agricultural and Food Chemistry. 2006;**54**(12):4168-4175. DOI: 10.1021/jf060224m

[34] Begić M, Oručević Žuljević S, Akagić A, Spaho N. Relationship between the physical and chemical quality parameters of common buckwheat (*Fagopyrum* Esculentum Moench) and tartary buckwheat (*Fagopyrum Tataricum* Moench). International Journal of Research in Agricultural Sciences. 2017;**4**(3):115-159

[35] Morishita T, Yamaguchi H, Degi K. The contribution of polyphenols to antioxidative activity in common buckwheat and tartary buckwheat grain. Plant Production Science. 2007;**10**(1):99-104. DOI: 10.1626/pps.10.99

[36] Patel K, Patel DK. The beneficial role of rutin, a naturally occurring flavonoid in health promotion and disease prevention: A systematic review and update. In: Watson RR, Preedy VR, editors. Bioactive Food as Dietary Interventions for Arthritis and Related Inflammatory Diseases. 2nd ed. Cambridge, MA: Academic Press; 2019. pp. 457-479

[37] Li S, Zhang QH. Advances in the development of functional foods from buckwheat. Critical Reviews in Food Science and Nutrition. 2001;**41**(6):451-464. DOI: 10.1080/20014091091887

[38] Liu B, Zhu Y. Extraction of flavonoids from flavonoid-rich parts in tartary buckwheat and identification of the main flavonoids. Journal of Food Engineering. 2007;**78**(2):584-587. DOI: 10.1016/j.jfoodeng.2005.11.001

[39] Afanas'ev IB, Dcrozhko AI, Brodskii AV, Kostyuk VA, Potapovitch AI. Chelating and free radical scavenging mechanisms of inhibitory action of rutin and quercetin in lipid peroxidation. Biochemical Pharmacology. 1989;**38**(11): 1763-1769. DOI: 10.1016/0006-2952(89) 90410-3

[40] Dietrych-Szostak D, Oleszek W. Effect of processing on the flavonoid content in buckwheat (*Fagopyrum esculentum* Möench) grain. Journal of Agricultural and Food Chemistry. 1999;**47**(10):4383-4387. DOI: 10.1021/jf990121m

[41] Kreft S, Knapp M, Kreft I. Extraction of rutin from buckwheat (*Fagopyrum esculentum* Moench) seeds and determination by capillary electrophoresis. Journal of Agricultural and Food Chemistry. 1999;**47**(11):2020-2023. DOI: 10.1021/jf990186p

[42] Park CH, Kim YB, Choi YS, Heo K, Kim SL, Lee KC, et al. Rutin content in food products processed from groats, leaves and flowers of buckwheat. Fagopyrum. 2000;**17**:63-66

[43] Zielińska D, Szawara-Nowak D, Zieliński H. Comparison of spectrophotometric and electrochemical methods for the evaluation of the antioxidant capacity of buckwheat products after hydrothermal treatment. Journal of Agricultural and Food Chemistry. 2007;**55**(15):6124-6131. DOI: 10.1021/jf071046f

[44] Zielińska D, Szawara-Nowak D, Zieliński H. Determination of the antioxidant activity of rutin and its contribution to the antioxidant capacity of diversified buckwheat origin material by updated analytical strategies. Polish Journal of Food and Nutrition Sciences. 2010;**60**(4):315-321

[45] Luthar Z, Zhou M, Golob A, Germ M. Breeding buckwheat for increased levels and improved quality of protein. Plants. 2021;**10**:14. DOI: 10.3390/plants10010014

[46] Fabjan N, Rode J, Kosir IJ, Wang Z, Zhang Z, Kreft I. Tartary buckwheat (*Fagopyrum tataricum* Gaertn.) as a source of dietary rutin and quercitrin. Journal of Agricultural and Food Chemistry. 2003;**51**(22):6452-6455. DOI: 10.1021/jf034543e

[47] Zielińska D, Zieliński H. Low molecular weight antioxidants and other biologically active components of buckwheat seeds. European Journal of Plant Science and Biotechnology. 2009;**3**:29-38

[48] Kim SJ, Maeda T, Sarker M, Takigawa S, MatsuuraEndo C, Yamauchi H, et al. Identification of anthocyanins in the sprouts of buckwheat. Journal of Agricultural and Food Chemistry. 2007;**55**(15):6314-6318. DOI: 10.1021/jf0704716

[49] Li D, Li X, Ding X. Composition and antioxidative properties of the flavonoid-rich fractions from tartary buckwheat grains. Food Science and Biotechnology. 2010;**19**(3):711-716

[50] Liu CL, Chen YS, Yang JH, Chiang BH. Antioxidant activity of tartary (*Fagopyrum tataricum* (L.) Gaertn.) and common (*Fagopyrum esculentum* Moench) buckwheat sprouts. Journal of Agricultural and Food Chemistry. 2008;**56**(1):173-178. DOI: 10.1021/jf072347s

[51] Liu JL, Tang Y, Xia ZM, Shao JR, Cai GZ, Luo Q. *Fagopyrum crispatifolium* J L. Liu, a new species of *Polygonaceae* from Sichuan. China. Journal of Systematic and Evolutionary. 2008;**46**:929-932

[52] Sharma S, Ali A, Ali J, Sahni JK, Baboota S. Rutin: Therapeutic potential and recent advances in drug delivery. Expert Opinion on Investigational Drugs. 2013;**22**(8):1063-1079. DOI: 10.1517/13543784.2013.805744

[53] Li L, Lietz G, Seal C. Buckwheat and CVD risk markers: A systematic review and meta-analysis. Nutrients. 2018;**10**(5):619. DOI: 10.3390/nu10050619

[54] Giménez-Bastida JA, Zieliński H. Buckwheat as a functional food and its effects on health. Journal of Agricultural and Food Chemistry. 2015;**63**(36):7896-7913. DOI: 10.1021/acs.jafc.5b02498

[55] Tambağ AK, Kazak F, Akalın PP, Kutlu T. The protective effect of rutin against methotrexate-induced nephrotoxicity in rats. Turkish Journal of Nephrology. 2021;**30**(3):218-223

[56] Jiang P, Burczynski F, Campbell C, Pierce G, Austria JA, Briggs CJ. Rutin and flavonoid in three buckwheat species Fagopyrum esculentum, F. tataricum, and F. *homotropicum* and their protective effects against lipid peroxidation. Food Research International. 2007;**40**(3):356-364. DOI: 10.1016/j.foodres.2006.10.009

[57] Yang N, Ren G. Application of near-infrared reflectance spectroscopy to the evaluation of rutin and D-chiro-inositol contents in Tartary Buckwheat. Journal of Agricultural and Food Chemistry. 2008;**56**(3):761-764. DOI: 10.1021/jf072453u

[58] Cai EP, Lin JK. Epigallocatechin gallate (EGCG) and rutin suppress the glucotoxicity through activating IRS2 and AMPK signaling in rat pancreatic β Cells. Journal of Agricultural and Food Chemistry. 2009;**57**(20):9817-9827. DOI: 10.1021/jf902618v

[59] Awatsuhara R, Harada K, Nomura T, Nikaido O, Nagao K. Alteration of antioxidative activity of rutin treated with food protein. Journal of Clinical Biochemistry and Nutrition. 2008;**43**:S512-S515

[60] Zielińska D, Turemko M, Kwiatkowski J, Zieliński H. Evaluation of flavonoid contents and antioxidant capacity of the aerial parts of common and tartary buckwheat plants. Molecules. 2012;**17**(8):9668-9682. DOI: 10.3390/molecules17089668

[61] Horbowicz M, Wiczkowski W, Koczkodaj D, Saniewski M. Effects of methyl jasmonate on accumulation of flavonoids in seedlings of common buckwheat (*Fagopyrum esculentum* Moench). Acta Biologica Hungarica. 2011;**62**(3):265-278. DOI: 10.1556/ABiol.62.2011.3.6

[62] Zhang R, Yao Y, Wang Y, Ren G. Antidiabetic activity of isoquercetin in diabetic KK-Ay mice. Nutrition and Metabolism. 2011;**8**:85. DOI: 10.1186/1743-7075-8-85

[63] Li Y, Duan S, Jia H, Bai C, Zhang L, Wang Z. Flavonoids from tartary buckwheat induce G2/M cell cycle arrest and apoptosis in human hepatoma HepG2 cells. Acta Biochim Biophys Sin. 2014;**46**(6):460-470. DOI: 10.1093/abbs/gmu023

[64] Li XH, Park NI, Xu H, Woo SH, Park CH, Park SU. Differential expression of flavonoid biosynthesis genes and accumulation of phenolic components in common buckwheat (*Fagopyrum esculentum*). Journal of

Agricultural and Food Chemistry. 2010;**58**(23):12176-12181. DOI: 10.1021/jf103310g

[65] Li YQ, Zhou FC, Gao F, Bian JS, Shan F. Comparative evaluation of quercetin, isoquercetin and rutin as inhibitors of α- glucosidase. Journal of Agricultural and Food Chemistry. 2009;**57**(24):11463-11468. DOI: 10.1021/jf903083h

[66] Agrawal PK, Chandan Agrawal C, Blunden G. Rutin: A potential antiviral for repurposing as a SARS-CoV-2 main protease (Mpro) inhibitor. Natural Product Communications. 2021;**16**(4):1-12. DOI: 10. 1177/ 1934 578X 21991723

[67] Rizzuti B, Grande F, Conforti F, Jimenez-Alesanco A, Ceballos-Laita L, Ortega-Alarcon D, et al. Rutin is a low micromolar inhibitor of SARS-CoV-2 main protease 3CLpro: Implications for drug design of quercetin analogs. Biomedicine. 2021;**9**:375. DOI: 10.3390/biomedicines9040375

[68] Watanabe M. Catechins as antioxidants from buckwheat (*Fagopyrum esculentum* Moench) groats. Journal of Agricultural and Food Chemistry. 1998;**46**(3):839-845. DOI: 10.1021/jf9707546

[69] Aleksenko SS. Antioxidant activity and phenolic components of buckwheat and barley by the data of spectrophotometry and HPLC. Journal of Analytical Chemistry. 2013;**68**(5):505-513. DOI: 10.1134/S106193481305002X

[70] Alonso-Amelot ME, Oliveros-Bastidas A, Calcagnopisarelli MP. Phenolics and condensed tannins of high altitude Pteridium arachnoideum in relation to sunlight exposure, elevation, and rain regime. Biochemical Systematics and Ecology. 2007;**35**(1):1-10. DOI: 10.1016/j.bse.2006.04.013

[71] Kishore G, Ranjan S, Pandey A, Gupta S. Influence of altitudinal variation on the antioxidant potential of tartar buckwheat of Western Himalaya. Food Science and Biotechnology. 2010;**19**:1355-1363. DOI: 10.1007/s10068-010-0193-9

[72] Mariotti M, Macchia M, Cerri D, Gatta D, Arduini I, Saccomanni G. Rutin content in the forage and grain of common buckwheat (*Fagopyrum esculentum*) as affected by sowing time and irrigation in a mediterranean environment. Crop and Pasture Science. 2020;**71**(2):171-182. DOI: 10.1071/CP19238

[73] Kalinova J, Triska J, Vrchotova N. Distribution of vitamin E, squalene, epicatechin, and rutin in common buckwheat plants (*Fagopyrum esculentum* Moench). Journal of Agricultural and Food Chemistry. 2006;**54**(15):5330-5335. DOI: 10.1021/jf060521r

[74] Guo XD, Ma YJ, Parry J, Gao JM, Yu LL, Wang M. Phenolics content and antioxidant activity of tartary buckwheat from different locations. Molecules. 2011;**16**(12):9850-9867. DOI: 10.3390/molecules16129850

[75] Sytar O. Phenolic acids in the inflorescences of different varieties of buckwheat and their antioxidant activity. Journal of King Saud University—Science. 2015;**24**(2):136-142. DOI: 10.1016/j.jksus.2014.07.001

[76] Bonafaccia G, Marocchini M, Kreft I. Composition and technological properties of the flour and bran from common and tartary buckwheat. Food Chemistry. 2003;**80**(1):9-15. DOI: 10.1016/S0308-8146(02)00228-5

[77] Giménez-Bastida JA, Piskula M, Zieliński H. Recent advances in development of gluten-free buckwheat products. Trends in Food Science and

Technology. 2015;**44**(1):58-65. DOI: 10.1016/j.tifs.2015.02.013

[78] Sedej I. Functional and antioxidant properties of new buckwheat products [thesis]. Serbia: Univerzitet u Novom Sadu. Tehnološki fakultet. 2011

[79] Kim SL, Kim SK, Park CH. Comparisons of lipid, fatty acids and tocopherols of different buckwheat species. Food Science and Biotechnology. 2002;**1**(4):332-336

[80] Zieliński H, Ciska E, Kozlowska H. The cereal grains: Focus on Vitamin E. Czech Journal of Food Sciences. 2001;**19**(5):182-188

[81] Alvarez-Jubete L, Holse M, Hansen Å, Arendt EK, Gallagher E. Impact of baking on vitamin E content of pseudocereals amaranth, quinoa, and buckwheat. Cereal Chemistry. 2009;**86**(5):511-515. DOI: 10.1094/CCHEM-86-5-0511

[82] Piironen V, Syväoja EL, Varo P, Salminen K, Koivistoinen P. Tocopherols and tocotrienols in cereal products from Finland. Cereal Chemistry. 1986;**63**: 78-81

[83] Horbowicz M, Brenac P, Obendorf RL. Fagopyritol B1, O-alpha-D-galactopyranosyl-(1→2)-Dchiro-inositol, a galactosyl cyclitol in maturing buckwheat seeds associated with desiccation tolerance. Planta. 1998;**205**(1):1-11. DOI: 10.1007/s004250050290

[84] Steadman KJ, Burgoon MS, Schuster RL, Lewis B, Edwardson SE, Obendorf RL. Fagopyritols, D-chiro-inositol, and other soluble carbohydrates in buckwheat seed milling fractions. Journal of Agricultural and Food Chemistry. 2000;**48**(7):2843-2847. DOI: 10.1021/jf990709t

[85] Steadman KJ, Fuller DJ, Obendorf RL. Purification and molecular structure of two digalactosyl D-chiro-inositols and two trigalactosyl D-chiro-inositols from buckwheat seeds. Carbohydrate Research. 2001;**331**(1):19-25. DOI: 10.1016/s0008-6215(00)00320-7

[86] Larner J, Huang LC, Schwartz CFW, Oswald AS, Shen TY, Kinter M, et al. Rat-liver insulin mediator which stimulates pyruvate-dehydrogenase phosphatase contains galactosamine and D-chiro-inositol. Biochemical and Biophysical Research Communications. 1988;**151**(3):1416-1426. DOI: 10.1016/s0006-291x(88)80520-5

[87] Obendorf RL, Horbowicz M, Ueda T, Steadman K. Fagopyritols: Occurrence, biosynthesis, analyses, and possible role. European Journal of Plant Science and Biotechnology. 2012;**6**:27-36

[88] Yao Y, Shan F, Bian J, Chen F, Wang M, Ren G. D-chiro-inositol-enriched tartary buckwheat bran extracts lowers the blood glucose level in KK-Ay mice. Journal of Agricultural and Food Chemistry. 2008;**56**(21):10027-10031. DOI: 10.1021/jf801879m

[89] Ortmeyer HK, Huang LC, Lu Z, Hansen BC, Larner J. Chiroinositol deficiency and insulin resistance. II. Acute effects of Dchiroinositol administration in streptozotocin-diabetic rats, normal rats given a glucose-load, and spontaneously insulin-resistant rhesusmonkeys. Endocrinology. 1993;**132**(2):646-651. DOI: 10.1210/en.132.2.646

[90] Ortmeyer HK, Larner J, Hansen BC. Effects of d-chiroinositol added to a meal on plasma glucose and insulin in hyperinsulinemic rhesus monkeys. Obesity Research. 1995;**3**(Suppl 4): 605S-608S. DOI: 10.1002/j.1550-8528.1995.tb00232.x

[91] Kalra B, Kalra S, Sharma JB. The inositols and polycystic ovary syndrome. Indian Journal of Endocrinology and Metabolism. 2016;**20**(5):720-724. DOI: 10.4103/2230-8210.189231

[92] Benelli E, Del Ghianda S, Di Cosmo C, Tonacchera M. A combined therapy with myo-inositol and D-chiro-inositol improves endocrine parameters and insulin resistance in PCOS young overweight women. International Journal of Endocrinology. 2016;**2016**:3204083. DOI: 10.1155/2016/3204083

[93] Kamenov Z, Gateva A. Inositols in PCOS. Molecules. 2020;**25**(23):5566. DOI: 10.3390/molecules25235566

[94] Normen L, Bryngelsson S, Johnsson M, Evheden P, Ellegard L, Brants H, et al. The phytosterol content of some cereal foods commonly consumed in Sweden and in the Netherlands. Journal of Food Composition and Analysis. 2002;**15**(6):693-704. DOI: 10.1006/jfca.2002.1098

[95] Dziedzic K, Kurek S, Mildner-Szkudlarz S, Kreft I, Walkowiak J. Fatty acids profile, sterols, tocopherol and squalene content in *Fagopyrum tataricum* seed milling fractions. Journal of Cereal Science. 2020;**96**:103118. DOI: 10.1016/j.jcs

[96] Amézqueta S, Galán E, Vila-Fernández I, Pumarola S, Carrascal M, Abian J, et al. The presence of d-fagomine in the human diet from buckwheat-based foodstuffs. Food Chemistry. 2013;**136**(3-4):1316-1321. DOI: 10.1016/j.foodchem.2012.09.038

[97] Gómez L, Molinar-Toribio E, Calvo-Torras MA, Adelantado C, Juan ME, Planas JM, et al. D-Fagomine lowers postprandial blood glucose and modulates bacterial adhesion. The British Journal of Nutrition. 2011;**107**(12):1739-1746. DOI: 10.1017/S00071145110 05009

[98] Amézqueta S, Galán E, Fuguet E, Carrascal M, Abián J, Torres JL. Determination of D-fagomine in buckwheat and mulberry by cation exchange HPLC/ESI–Q-MS. Analytical and Bioanalytical Chemistry. 2012;**402**(5):1953-1960. DOI: 10.1007/s00216-011-5639-2

[99] Peng L-X, Wang J-B, Hu L-X, Zhao J-L, Xiang D-B, Zou L, et al. Rapid and simple method for the determination of emodin in tartary buckwheat (*Fagopyrum tataricum*) by high-performance liquid chromatography coupled to a diode array detector. Journal of Agricultural and Food Chemistry. 2013;**61**(4):854-857. DOI: 10.1021/jf304804c

[100] Izhaki I. Emodin—A secondary metabolite with multiple ecological functions in higher plants. The New Phytologist. 2002;**155**(2):205-217. DOI: 10.1046/j.1469-8137.2002.00459.x

[101] Amarowicz R, Dykes GA, Pegg RB. Antibacterial activity of tannin constituents from Phaseolus vulgaris, Fagoypyrum esculentum, Corylus avellana and Juglans nigra. Fitoterapia. 2008;**9**(3):217-221. DOI: 10.1016/j.fitote.2007.11.019

[102] Miyake K, Morita R, Handoyo T, Maeda T, Morita N. Characterization of graded buckwheat flours and some properties of germinated 'Mancan' buckwheat grains. Fagopyrum. 2004;**21**:91-97

[103] Aoyagi Y. An angiotensin-I converting enzyme inhibitor from buckwheat (*Fagopyrum esculentum* Moench) flour. Phytochemistry. 2006;**67**(6):618-621. DOI: 10.1016/j.phytochem.2005.12.022

[104] Maejima Y, Nakatsugawa H, Ichida D, Maejim M, Aoyagi Y, Maoka T, et al. Functional components in fermented buckwheat sprouts. Bioscience, Biotechnology, and Biochemistry. 2011;**75**:1708-1712. DOI: 10.1271/bbb.110241

[105] Suzuki T, Watanabe M, Iki M, Aoyagi Y, Kim SJ, Mukasa Y, et al. Time-course study and effects of drying method on concentrations of γ-aminobutyric acid, flavonoids, anthocyanin, and 2′′ hydroxynicotianamine in leaves of buckwheats. Journal of Agricultural and Food Chemistry. 2009;**57**(1):259-264. DOI: 10.1021/jf802731d

[106] Hung P, Morita N. Distribution of phenolic components in the graded flours milled from whole buckwheat grains and their antioxidant capacities. Food Chemistry. 2008;**109**(2):325-331. DOI: 10.1016/j.foodchem.2007.12.060

[107] Inglett GA, Chen D, Berhow M, Lee S. Antioxidant activity of commercial buckwheat flours and their free and bound phenolic compositions. Food Chemistry. 2011;**125**(3):923-929. DOI: 10.1016/j.foodchem.2010.09.076

[108] Gallardo C, Jiménez L, García-Conesa M-T. Hydroxycinnamic acid composition and in vitro antioxidant activity of selected grain fractions. Food Chemistry. 2006;**99**(3):455-463. DOI: 10.1016/j.foodchem.2005.07.053

[109] Chen XW, Chen YJ, Li JY, Wang YH, Yang XQ. Enzyme-assisted development of biofunctional polyphenol-enriched buckwheat protein: Physicochemical properties, in vitro digestibility, and antioxidant activity. Journal of the Science of Food and Agriculture. 2019;**99**(6):3176-3185. DOI: 10.1002/jsfa.9534

[110] Ge RH, Wang H. Nutrient components and bioactive components in tartary buckwheat bran and flour as affected by thermal processing. International Journal of Food Properties. 2020;**23**(1):127-137. DOI: 10.1080/10942912.2020.1713151

[111] Džafić A, Oručević S, Šehovac F, Melezović T, Berbić N. Granulation of common and tatrary buckwheat at wholemeal flour and its effect on physical properties of flour. Works of Faculty of Agriculture and Food Sciences University of Sarajevo. 2014;**64**(2):91-99

[112] Chandrssekaran S, Ramanathan S, Basak T. Microwave food processing—A review. Food Research International. 2013;**52**(1):234-261. DOI: 10.1016/j.foodres.2013.02.033

[113] Suzuki T, Yutaka H, Funatsuki W, Nakatsuka K. Purification and characterization of flavonol 3-glucosidase, and its activity during ripening in tartary buckwheat seeds. Plant Science. 2002;**163**(3):417-423. DOI: 10.1016/S0168-9452(02)00158-9

[114] Vogrinćić M, Timoracka M, Melichacova S, Vollmannova A, Kreft I. Degradation of rutin and polyphenols during the preparation of tartary buckwheat bread. Journal of the Science of Food and Agriculture. 2010;**58**(8):4883-4887. DOI: 10.1021/jf9045733

[115] Sakač M, Torbica A, Sedej I, Hadnađev M. Influence of breadmaking on antioxidant capacity of gluten free breads based on rice and buckwheat flours. Food Research International. 2011;**44**(9):2806-2813. DOI: 10.1016/j.foodres.2011.06.026

[116] Chlopicka J, Pasko P, Gorinstein S, Jedryas A, Zagrodzki P. Total phenolic and total flavonoid content, antioxidant activity and sensory evaluation of pseudocereal breads. LWT-Food Science

and Technology. 2012;**46**(2):548-555. DOI: 10.1016/j.lwt.2011.11.009

[117] Verardo V, Arrárez-Román D, Segura-Carretero A, Marconi E, Fernández-Gutíerrez A, Fiorenza CM. Determination of free and bound phenolic components in buckwheat spaghetti by RP-HPLC-ESI-TOF-MS: Effect of thermal processing from farm to fork. Journal of Agricultural and Food Chemistry. 2011;**59**(14):7700-7707. DOI: 10.1021/jf201069k

[118] Biney K, Beta T. Phenolic profile and carbohydrate digestibility of durum spaghetti enriched with buckwheat flour and bran. LWT—Food Science and Technology. 2014;**57**(2):569-579. DOI: 10.1016/j.lwt.2014.02.033

[119] Jambrec DJ, Mišan A, Pestorić MV, Psodorov ĐB, Mandić AI, Sakač MB, et al. Functional and sensory properties of pasta enriched with light buckwheat flour. In: Proceeding of the 6ths Central European Congress on Food, CEFood. Novi Sad, Serbia: EFFoST (European Federation of Food Science and Technology), IUFoST (International Union of Food Science and Technology), CEI (Central European Initiative); 2012. pp. 1-6

[120] Jambrec D, Sakač M, Mišan A, Mandić A, Pestorić M. Effect of autoclaving and cooking on phenolic components in buckwheat-enriched whole wheat tagliatelle. Journal of Cereal Science. 2015;**66**:1-9. DOI: 10.1016/j.jcs.2015.09.004

[121] Cho YJ, Lee S. Extraction of rutin from tartary buckwheat milling fractions and evaluation of its thermal stability in an instant fried noodle system. Food Chemistry. 2015;**176**:40-44. DOI: 10.1016/j.foodchem.2014.12.020

[122] Randhir R, Kwon Y-I, Shetty K. Effect of thermal processing on phenolics, antioxidant activity and health-relevant functionality of select grain sprouts and seedlings. Innovative Food Science and Emerging Technologies. 2008;**9**(3):355-364. DOI: 10.1016/j.ifset.2007.10.004

[123] Zieliński H, Michalska A, Piskula MK, Kozlowska H. Antioxidants in thermally treated buckwheat groats. Molecular Nutrition and Food Research. 2006;**50**(9):824-832. DOI: 10.1002/mnfr.200500258

[124] Hęś M, Dziedzic K, Górecka D, Drożdżyńska A, Gujska E. Effect of boiling in water of barley and buckwheat groats on the antioxidant properties and dietary fiber composition. Plant Foods for Human Nutrition. 2014;**69**(3):276-282. DOI: 10.1007/s11130-014-0425-x

[125] Zieliński H, Michalska A, Amigo-Benavente M, Del Castillo D, Piskuła MK. Changes in protein quality and antioxidant properties of buckwheat seeds and groats induced by roasting. Journal of Agricultural and Food Chemistry. 2009;**57**(11):4771-4776. DOI: 10.1021/jf900313e

[126] Zhang M, Chen H, Li J, Pei Y, Liang Y. Antioxidant properties of tartary buckwheat extracts as affected by different thermal processing methods. LWT—Food Science and Technology. 2010;**43**(1):181-185. DOI: 10.1016/j.lwt.2009.06.020

[127] Costantini L, Lukšič L, Molinari R, Kreft I, Bonafaccia G, Manzi L, et al. Development of gluten-free bread using tartary buckwheat and chia flour rich in flavonoids and omega-3 fatty acids as ingredients. Food Chemistry. 2014;**15**(165):232-340. DOI: 10.1016/j.foodchem.2014.05.095

[128] Delgado-Andrade C. Maillard reaction products: Some considerations

on their health effects. Clinical Chemistry and Laboratory Medicine. 2014;**52**(1):53-60. DOI: 10.1515/cclm-2012-0823

[129] Norton T, Sun D-W. Recent advances in the use of high pressure as an effective processing technique in the food industry. Food and Bioprocess Technology. 2008;**1**:2-34. DOI: 10.1007/s11947-007-0007-0

[130] Błaszczak W, Zielińska D, Zieliński H, Szawara-Nowak D, Fornal J. Antioxidant properties and rutin content of high pressure-treated raw and roasted buckwheat groats. Food and Bioprocess Technology. 2013;**6**:92-100. DOI: 10.1007/s11947-011-0669-5

[131] Zhou Z, Ren X, Wang F, Li J, Si X, Cao R, et al. High pressure processing manipulated buckwheat antioxidant activity, anti-adipogenic properties and starch digestibility. Journal of Cereal Science. 2015;**66**:31-36. DOI: 10.1016/j.jcs.2015.09.002

[132] Hayashi T, Takahashi Y, Todoriki S. Sterilization of foods with low-energy electrons ("soft-electrons"). Radiation Physics and Chemistry. 1998;**52**:1-6. DOI: 10.1016/S0969-806X(98)00077-2

[133] Chun HH, Song KB. Optimisation of the combined treatments of aqueous chlorine dioxide, fumaric acid and ultravioletC for improving the microbial quality and maintaining sensory quality of common buckwheat sprout. International Journal of Food Science and Technology. 2013;**49**(1):121-127. DOI: 10.1111/ijfs.12283

[134] Orsák M, Lachman J, Vejdová M, Pivec V, Hamouz K. Changes of selected secondary metabolites in potatoes and buckwheat caused by UV, gamma- and microwave irradiation. Rostlinna Vyroba. 2001;**47**(11):493-500

[135] Hossen Z. Light emitting diodes increase phenolics of buckwheat (*Fagopyrum esculentum*) sprouts. Journal of Plant Interactions. 2007;**2**:71-78. DOI: 10.1080/17429140701288228

[136] Tabaković M, Simić M, Stanisavljević R, Sečanski M, Lj Ž, Štrbanović R. Buckwheat seed quality during the five-year storage in various packing materials. Plant, Soil and Environment. 2019;**65**(7):349-354. DOI: 10.17221/237/2019-PSE

Chapter 7

Nutritional Value, Methods for Extraction and Bioactive Compounds of Quinoa

Luis Olivera, Ivan Best, Perla Paredes, Neyma Perez, Luis Chong and Alejandro Marzano

Abstract

Quinoa (*Chenopodium quinoa* Willd.) is a crop belonging to the Chenopodiaceae family that originated in the high Andean region of South America. Currently, the main producers of quinoa are Bolivia and Peru; this crop groups around 250 species and 3000 varieties. It has a high adaptability, which allows it to be cultivated in cold climates in the high Andean regions, as well as in subtropical conditions, and grows from sea level to more than 4000 meters above sea level. Due to its high nutritional value and nutritional properties, quinoa is considered "one of the grains of the 21st century." It is high in protein without gluten, polyunsaturated fatty acids, carbohydrates, vitamins, minerals, and fiber, as well as high levels of bioactive compounds such as flavonoids, phenolic acids, bioactive peptides, phytosteroid betalains, phytosterols, and saponins. From quinoa, a protein concentrate of high biological value can be extracted due to its content of the nine essential amino acids, as well as an oil with high antioxidant activity due to its high levels of tocopherols. These by-products have a high economic and commercial value and can be produced on an industrial scale for use in the food, cosmetic, and pharmaceutical industries.

Keywords: *Chenopodium quinoa*, Andean region, phenolic compounds, essential amino acids, antioxidant activity

1. Introduction

Quinoa is a plant of the *Chenopodium* genus original from South America and well distributed in countries that belonged to the Inca empire, located on the Andean mountain range, from southern Colombia through Ecuador, Peru, Bolivia, and up to northern Chile [1]. It is considered one of the oldest crops in the Americas. Archeological findings in Chile have shown that quinoa was cultivated around 3000 B. C. In the case of Peru, in Ayacucho, it has been shown that quinoa was cultivated before 5000 B.C. [2]. It has a great edaphological and climatic adaptability and grows at different altitudes, from sea level to the altitude of the Bolivian altiplano withstand low temperatures down to −8.0°C, alkaline soils (pH 8), and salinity of 52 mS/cm, which has allowed the expansion of large cultivation areas in different geographical areas, thus promoting the exploitation of its diverse nutritional and pharmacological properties [3]. The main survival mechanism of quinoa against frost is to avoid the formation of ice by an internal reduction in temperature. Quinoa has a high soluble sugar content that can cause decrease of the freezing point and therefore the lethal temperature of the leaf tissue [4]. It is designated as a "pseudocereal" and even as an oleaginous " pseudocereal" [5], and due to its characteristic of resistance and tolerance to stress and its nutritional and biological properties, quinoa has been described as "one of the grains of the 21st century" [6].

2. Botanical aspects

Quinoa was initially classified based on the color of the plant and its fruits and then based on the morphological types of the plant. Although due to a wide variation observed, quinoa has been classified as a race. Quinoa from Bolivia, Peru, and Ecuador has been classified into 17 races. Thus, one of the most useful classifications is the one that describes five ecotypes: sea level, valley, subtropical, salt flat, and altiplano [2]. Other authors [7, 8] mention that quinoa has the following systematic classification:

Kingdom: Plantae,
Division: Magnoliophyta.
Class: Magnoliopsida.
Order: Caryophyllales.
Family: Amaranthaceae.
Subfamily: Chenopodiaceae.
Genus: Chenopodium.
Species: C. quinoa Willdenow.
Common name: Quinoa.

Although the name quinoa is the most widespread, there are numerous names used by different ethnic groups in the vast production territory; for example, arrocillo, Inca wheat, in some parts of Peru.

The annual herbaceous plant has an average height between 1.0 and 3.0 m depending on the variety and planting density; its central stem is woody and can be branched or unbranched (**Figure 1A**), also varying in color (green, red, or purple); its roots can reach up to 30 cm depending on the depth of planting. Leaves are formed by the petiole and lamina, are rich in calcium and oxalate crystals that reduce excessive transpiration allowing the maintenance of adequate humidity inside the plant. The color is very variable, ranging from green in young plants to red or violet with different shades in more mature plants [10]. In many areas of the Andean region, the young leaves before flowering are suitable for human consumption due to their high nutritional value attributed to their vitamin, mineral, and protein content. The panicle appears from the leaf axil along the stem or may arise from the top of the plant (**Figure 1B**); the flowers are self-fertilized, although it can also be produced by cross-pollination [8]. The seeds are small, round, and flat with a length of 2.5 mm and 1.0 mm in diameter (**Figure 1C**); seed colors can vary from white to gray and black, or it can be yellow and red. Seeds have three main components: embryo, perisperm, and episperm. Embryo is formed by two cotyledons and constitutes 30% of the total volume of the seed and contains between 35 and 40% of the total seed protein.

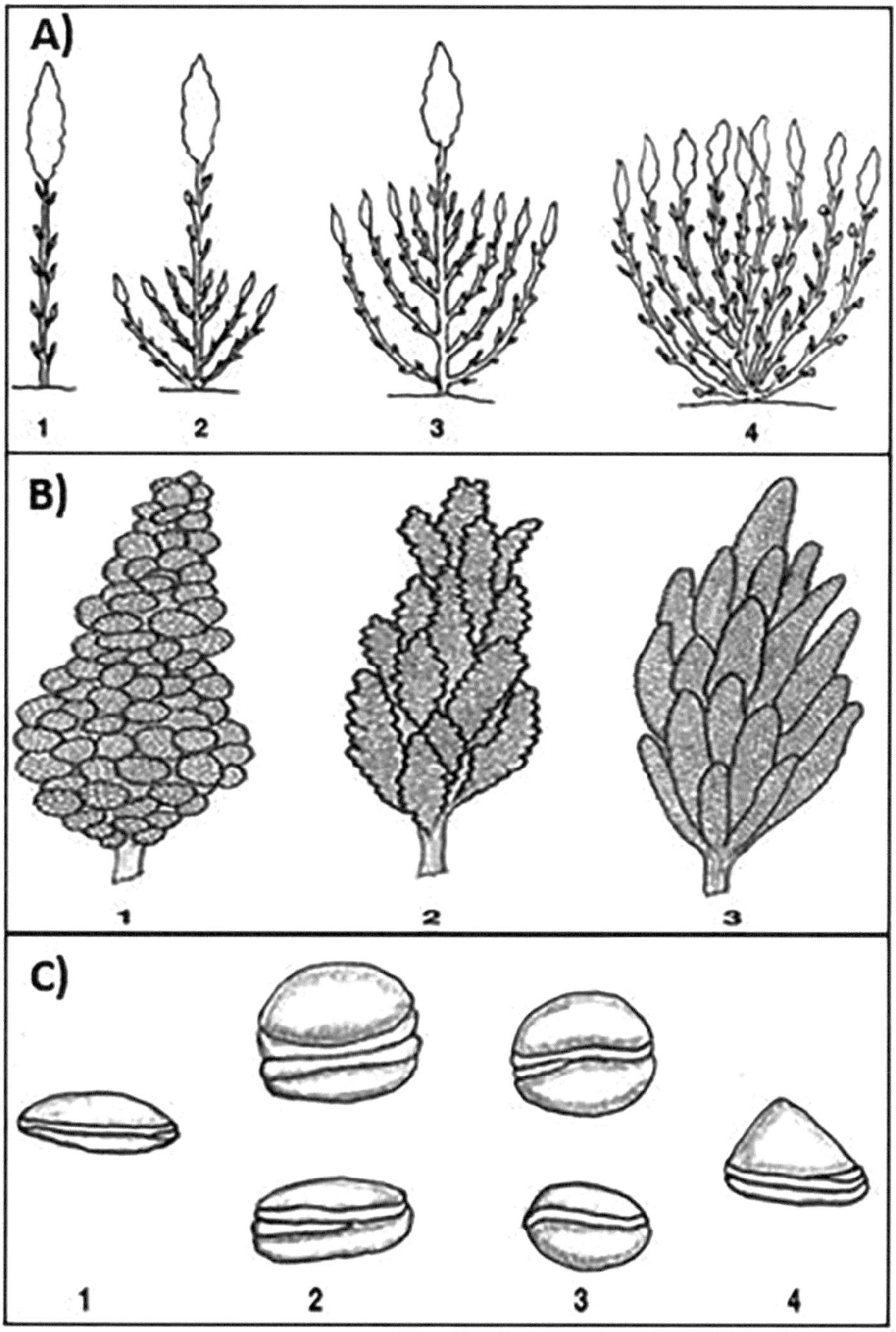

Figure 1.
Characterization of the quinoa plant. A. Growth habit: (1) Simple, (2) Branched to the lower third, (3) Branched to the second third, (4) Branched with undefined main panicle; B. Panicle shape: (1) Glomerulate, (2) Intermediate, (3) Amarantiform; C. Grain shape: (1) Lenticular, (2) Cylindrical, (3) Ellipsoidal, (4) Conical [9].

Perisperm represents almost 60% of the seed surface and contains only 6.3–8.3% of the total proteins. Pericarp contains the saponins that give the characteristic bitter taste to the seed [11].

3. Production

Countries with the highest production of quinoa are Bolivia and Peru, which account for more than 90% of total world production [12]. Until 2000, world quinoa production did not exceed approximately 50,000 metric tons (t) per year. From 2003 to 2018, quinoa production in the Andean region has increased by about 165,000 t (**Figure 2A**). This growth has made it possible to meet export demand, and more than half of the quinoa produced in South America (Peru, Bolivia, and Ecuador) is exported mostly to the United States and Europe. In an average of 30 years (1983–2013), the yield in Bolivia was 0.55 tons per hectare (t/ha) with a range of 0.43–0.68 t/ha. In Peru from 2007 to 2014, yield efficiencies have doubled from 0.97 to 1.93 t/ha; being as of 2018, the average yield in the region of 1 t/ ha (**Figure 2B**) [13].

Cropland has increased significantly. Bolivia increased more than four times in the last 30 years. Since 2007, harvested areas have increased from 32,959 to 55,000 ha in Peru. In Latin American Peru, Bolivia, and Ecuador recorded a total of 172,000 ha harvested in 2018. In these three countries, quinoa is produced under diverse agro-ecological conditions and production systems. Traditional production systems are characterized by medium plots (up to 10 ha) and small scale (<2 ha) with low input technology [13]. Production costs for Peruvian quinoa are $2200 USD/t, and farm gate prices range from $4000–4500 USD/t (conventional) to $5200 USD/t (organic) [12].

4. Composition and nutritional value

Quinoa is rich in protein, lipids, fiber, vitamins, and minerals. The grain contains an excellent nutritional profile (**Table 1**), starch (32–60%), protein (10–18%), fat (4.4–8.8%), fiber (1.1% and 13.4%), ash (2.3–3.7%), formed mainly from potassium and phosphorus [18, 19]. Quinoa also contains a high amount of vitamin B and vitamin E.

4.1 Protein

The average protein content is higher (12 to 23%), compared with other grains such as barley (11% dry basis), rice (7.5% dry basis) or corn (13.3% dry basis), and is comparable to wheat (15.4% dry basis) [14]. The proteins present in quinoa are of high quality, including albumins (35%) and globulins (37%) and, to a lesser extent, prolamins. The quality of these proteins is comparable to the protein present in milk (casein) [8]. It contains all the essential amino (**Table 2**), which is why it is considered a complete food [23], and it is also low in prolamine (0.5–7.0%), indicating that it is not allergenic [24].

4.2 Lipids

The fat content in quinoa seeds averages 2–10% and is considered as an alternative to oilseeds due to its lipid composition. Triglycerides are the main fraction of fats and constitute more than half of the neutral lipids [25]. Quinoa and soybean oils present a very similar fatty acid composition, with linolenic acid (18: 2n-6: 52%) and linolenic acid (18, 3n-6: 40%) being the most representative (**Table 3**) [27]. Quinoa oil has a high antioxidant quality, a high content of polyunsaturated fatty acids including

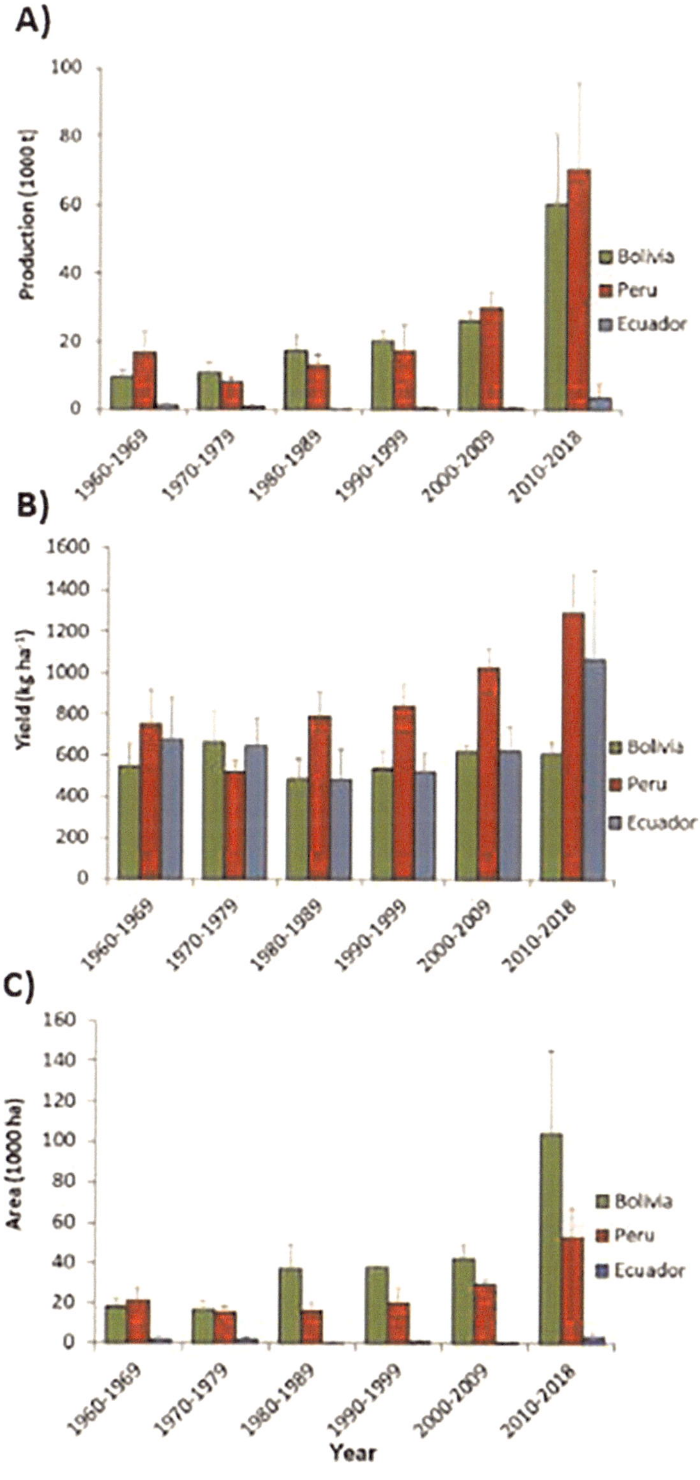

Figure 2.
Dynamics of quinoa production (A), yield (B), and area (C) in three countries of the Andean region between 1961 and 2018 [13].

Components	Jancurová et al. [2]	Hussain et al. [8]	Vilcacundo & Hernández-Ledesma [6]	Abugoch James [14]	Wright et al. [15]	Bruin [16]	Lalaleo et al. [17]
Protein	16,5	10–18	13,1–16,7	12–23	16,7	15,6	12,5
Fat	6,3	4,4–8,8	5,5–7,6	1,8–9,5	5,5	7,4	8,5
Fiber	3,8	1,1–13,4	7–11,7	7–9,7	10,5	2,9	1,92
Ashes	3,8	2,4–3,7	ND	ND	3,8	3,2	3,7
Carbohydrates	69,0	32–60	32–69	32–69,2	74.7	69,7	60,0
Kcal /100 g	399	ND	ND	ND	ND	ND	ND

ND, not detected.

Table 1.
Chemical composition of quinoa (g /100 g dry weight).

Amino acid	Kozioł [20]	Dini et al. [21]	Repo-Carrasco et al. [22]	Wright et al. [15]
Histidine	3.2	2,0	2,7	3,1
Isoleucine	4,4	7,4	3,4	3,3
Leucine	6,6	6,1	6,1	5,8
Methionine + cysteine	4,8	4,5	4,8	2,0
Phenylalanine + Tyrosine	7,3	7,5	6,2	6,2
Threonine	3,8	3,5	3,4	2,5
Valine	4,5	6,0	4,2	4,0
Lysine	6,1	4,6	5,6	6,1
Tryptophan	1,2	ND	1,1	ND

ND, not detected.

Table 2.
Essential amino acid profile (g protein/100 g).

Fatty acid	Abugoch James [14]	Kozioł [20]	Repo-Carrasco et al. [22]	Ruales & Nair [26]
Oleic C18:1	22,8–29,5	23,3	26,0	24,8
Linoleic C18:2 (n-6)	48,1–52,3	53,1	50,2	52,3
Linolenic C18:3 (n-3)	4,6–8	6,2	4,8	3,9

Table 3.
Saturated fatty acid (g/100 g of oil extract).

omega-3 and omega-6 fatty acids (63% of the total), and a significant amount of tocopherols (2.5 mg/g oil) [28]. On the other hand, linoleic acid is metabolized to arachidonic acid and linolenic acid to eicosapentaenoic acid (EPA) and docosahexaenoic acid (DHA) [29]. Polar lipids account for about 25% of the total, composed mainly of phospholipids (lysophosphatidylethanolamine and choline), of the neutral lipids (glycerides and sterols), triglycerides account for 74% and diglycerides for 20%, while monoglycerides and waxes account for 3% [8].

4.3 Carbohydrates

Quinoa has a significant amount of carbohydrates and represents between 67% and 74%, of which starch is the most important carbohydrate and represents approximately 58.1–64.2% of dry matter, variation of which is attributed to differences in genotypes and growing conditions [24]. Its granules have a polygonal shape with a diameter of 2 μm, being smaller than those of common cereals. Due to its size, it can be used as a biodegradable filler in polymer containers [23]. It is also an ideal thickener for frozen foods and other applications where resistance to retrogradation is desired, because of its freeze–thaw stability [30]. Carbohydrates include amylose with a content of about 11%, and other carbohydrates, which have been documented, include monosaccharides (2%) and disaccharides (2.3%), crude fiber (2.5–3.9%), and marshmallows (2.9–3.6%) [27]. Sucrose is also present in significant amounts compared with other sugars [23]. It contains a low proportion of glucose (19.0 mg/100 g) and fructose (19.6 mg/100 g). This is important in the fermentation of malted beverages [31].

4.4 Fiber

Quinoa is considered an important source of dietary fiber accounting for about 2.6–10% of the total dietary fiber weight. Approximately 78% of the amount of fiber in quinoa is insoluble and 22% in soluble form [24]. Although washing and abrasion processes are performed to remove saponins, this does not influence the fiber content [25]. Research reports that the dietary fiber content of quinoa is equal to that of other cereals and grains. Although, the fiber composition of quinoa is different from other cereals, biochemistry and therapeutics are still important to study the potential of quinoa and thus understand its specific physiological impact [8].

4.5 Minerals

Quinoa has a high content of calcium, iron, magnesium, iron, copper, and zinc (**Table 4**), covering the amounts needed to maintain a balanced human diet of calcium, phosphorus, potassium, and magnesium of 874, 2735.0–4543.3, 9562.2, and 1901.5 mg/kg, respectively [24]. In general, many of these minerals are higher than those reported for most cereal crops such as barley oats, rice, maize, or wheat [23].

4.6 Vitamins

The vitamin content of quinoa is interesting. It has high levels of vitamin B6 and total folate, whose amounts can cover the daily requirement of children and adults, as for riboflavin content, 100 g provides 80% of the daily needs of children and 40% of adults [14]. The niacin content does not cover the daily requirement; however, it is beneficial for the diet, the values of thiamine in quinoa are lower than those of oats and barley, but those of niacin, riboflavin, vitamin B6, and total folate are higher (**Table 5**).

Minerals	Kozioł [20]	Repo-Carrasco et al. [22]	Ruales & Nair [26]	Bhargava et al. [32]	KONISHI et al. [33]	Dini et al. [21]
Ca	1487	940	874	1274	863	275
P	3837	1400	5300	3869	4110	4244
Mg	2496	2700	260	ND	5020	ND
Fe	132	168	81	20	150	26
Zn	44	48	36	48	40	27.5
K	9267	ND	12,000	6967	7320	75
Cu	51	37	10	ND	ND	ND

ND, not detected.

Table 4.
Mineral composition (mg/ kg dry weight).

Vitaminas	Kozioł [20]	Ruales & Nair [26]
ácido ascórbico	4	16,4
α−tocoferol	5,37	2,6
Tiamina (B1)	0,38	0,4
Riboflavina (B2)	0,39	ND
Niacina B3	1,06	ND

ND, not detected.

Table 5.
Concentration of vitamins (mg/100 g dry weight).

5. Processed uses and current situation

At present, the processed uses given to quinoa are mainly from the flour obtained from it, which can replace that of corn and wheat, since various levels of quinoa flour substitution have been reported, for example, in sweet biscuits (60% quinoa), in noodles and pasta (30–40%), and in bread (10–13%) [27]. Other uses or innovations include quinoa beer that meets the sensory acceptance requirements, reaching a high alcoholic content (between 48 and 74°GL) and for the production of chocolates with quinoa filling with good physicochemical, organoleptic, microbiological, and nutritional characteristics [34].

There are other potential products derived from quinoa, which are obtained by extracting compounds from quinoa and for the creation of value-added products. Examples of these products are oil extraction, protein concentrates and isolates, starches, bioactive compounds, among others, for use in the food and pharmaceutical industry (**Table 6**, [35]). Compared with the starch content of wheat and barley, quinoa starch has a higher viscosity, greater water retention, and expansion capacity, as well as a higher gelatinization temperature, which translates into better performance as a thickening agent. Due to these properties, quinoa starch is very suitable for the production of prepared frozen baby foods, as it shows good freeze–thaw stability [36]. Due to its protein and starch content, quinoa can be used for the production of

Quinoa-derived product	Production method	Uses
Treated seeds	Superheated steam treatment to expand the seeds and reduce cooking time. Mechanical abrasion, washing, or a combination to debitter seeds.	Superheated steam treatment to expand the seeds and reduce cooking time. Mechanical abrasion, washing, or a combination to debitter seeds
Beverages	Seeds are soaked, malted, kilned, mashed, cooled, and fermented with yeast	Gluten-free fermented alcoholic beverage
	Mixing of quinoa extract, tiger nut (Cyperus esculentus), and α-amylases for hydrolysis of starches to thermostable maltodextrin within a beverage formulation.	Substitute for animal or plantderived milk
Protein concentrate	Extraction and precipitation *via* alkali or enzyme treatment	Used in foods, animal food, or sports performance and recovery
Lipid	Extraction and molecular distillation to obtain a refined oil	Dermatological use
Carbohydrate	Extraction of maltodextrin via alkali or enzyme treatment of quinoa flour to produce a gel-form to deliver quinoaderived peptides. Use of quinoa starches of specific shape and particle size	Cream substitute that mimics the mouth feel of fat/cream in food

Table 6.
Uses and processing methods.

edible films and as an emulsion stabilizing agent, specifically for Pickering emulsions [37]. Even incorporation of quinoa into food products has been shown to help extend shelf life and reduce microbial spoilage of food products.

6. Saponins

Saponins are secondary metabolites or glycoside compounds that form the family of compounds structurally constituted by steroids (C27) or triterpenoids (C30) [27]. **Figure 3** presents an amphiphilic character [39]. Saponins are found in the pericarp or

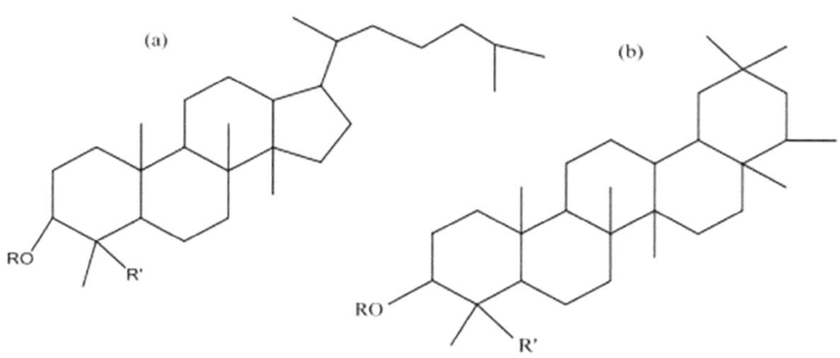

Figure 3.
Structures of sapogenins: steroid (a) and triterpenoid (b) [38].

outer part of the seed, interfering with its palatability and digestibility, making it necessary to eliminate them before consumption, as well as imparting a bitter taste and tending to foam in aqueous solutions [2]. Bitter taste can be easily separated from the seed either by the wet method, i.e., by rinsing the seed in cold alkaline water or by the dry method, i.e., by roasting and then rubbing the grains to remove the outer layers [40]; however, both methods do not achieve the total removal of saponins, so it is necessary to develop new methods of saponin removal from quinoa seeds.

The amount of saponins present in quinoa seeds depends on the variety so the content in bitter genotypes varies from 140 to 2300 mg/100 g dry weight, while on sweet genotypes ranges from 20 to 40 mg/100 g dry weight [40]. Up to 87 complex triterpene saponins from the quinoa seed coat have been identified [41] as well as the transcription factor involved in the control of seed triterpene saponin synthesis has also been identified [42], so it is expected that this finding will allow progress in the selection of sweet quinoa varieties with low saponin content.

Chemistry and pharmacological studies of properties of saponins documented that saponins possess many biological properties in which their analgesic, antiviral, antimicrobial cytotoxic, antifungal, anti-inflammatory, hypocholesterolemic, surfactant, antioxidant, hemolytic, immunoadjuvant, antiadipogenic, and molluscicidal activities stand out [1, 42]. These properties are of utmost importance as they can be processed and by-products are obtained for the food, cosmetic, and pharmaceutical industries [43]. Saponin possesses natural surfactants, which can lower the surface tension forming foams at the time of agitation and thus forms colloidal solutions, and soaps, creams, detergents, and shampoos can be obtained [44]. On the other hand, research has shown that saponins are good fungicides because they can control phytopathogenic fungal pests [45].

7. Bioactive compounds of quinoa

According to Melini, V. & Melini, F. (2021), through a systematic review, they show that the most sought-after and investigated functional compounds in quinoa seeds are phenolic compounds, of which flavonoids are the most studied while flavonodes and isoflavones have been studied on a smaller scale. Furthermore, only three studies have been reported for hydrophilic betalains. Additionally, among the lipophilic functional components, the most studied are the tocal ones, followed by the carotenoids [46].

Functional components of quinoa seed.

To begin with, the functional components have a great diversity of molecules that can modulate one to more metabolic processes in humans. In addition, they can be hydrophilic, of which we have phenolic compounds and betalains, or lipophilic; there are carotenoids, tocoles, and phytoecdysteorids [46].

7.1 Hydrophilic compounds

7.1.1 Phenolic compounds

They are secondary plant metabolites that have a variety of chemical structures that have in common the presence of one or more hydroxyl groups on aromatic rings. On the other hand, the different results of the detection of phenolic compounds in quinoa seeds in the world, in the first place, are that the crops analyzed in China were of a white and pigmented variety, where the grain was subjected to grinding to observe to what extent this can affect the content of these components; it is known that phenolic compounds are present in the outer layers of the grain, where the total phenolic content of the pigmented varieties were 2–3 times higher than white varieties. This difference in phenolic content may be due to the fact that the genotypes are different and the different pedoclimatic conditions, thus being the crops from China those that had high phenolic content compared with other parts of Asia [46]. On the other hand, studies of samples from Peru, Chile, Brazil, Argentina, and Colombia were carried out; where the free phenolic content was made in quinoa grown in Peru and Chile, where quinoa grown in Peru showed higher values than those of Chile. Finally, flavonoids have been found in samples of quinoa from Peru, the United States, and Korea, with Peru having a higher total flavonoid content than the others. However, other studies show that Korean crops have a higher content of total flavonoids than the Peruvian culture [46].

7.1.2 Betalains

They are pigments that are soluble in water and are responsible for the color of plant tissues; they can be classified into betacyanins and bexanthins [46]. Regarding the content of betalains in quinoa, the content of betalains has been determined in quinoa samples from the Peruvian highlands, where values that are in the range of 0.15 and 6.10 mg have been found. In several betalains, proline-derived betaxanthin was found in varieties with light yellow seeds and only in a black variety [46].

7.2 Lipophilic compounds

7.2.1 Carotenoids

Also known as natural pigments that give a yellow to orange-red color to plant tissue. We also find carotents and xanthophylls as major subgroups of carotenoids [46]. Additionally, the consumption of carotenoids has beneficial effects for human health such as protection against cardiovascular diseases, cataracts, cancer, and muscle degeneration [46].

On the other hand, regarding the content of carotenoids, they have been studied in samples of quinoa grown in Egypt and Finland, as in commercial samples, where B-carotene and lycopene were found in five genotypes of quinoa grown in Egypt, also B-carotene could be found in a commercial white quinoa sample, but high levels were found in pigmented quinoa sample. Furthermore, regarding the Finnish sample, six carotenoids were found in quinoa samples [46].

7.2.2 Tocoles

They are methylated phenols with a saturated side chain; in addition, tocopherols exist in four isoforms, α-, β-, γ-, and δ-tocopherol differing in the position of the methyl group on the chromanol ring [46]. On the other hand, the tocol content has been moderately investigated in quinoa seeds, carrying out a study of four varieties of quinoa grown in Peru, where the main isomer of tocopherol was α-tocopherol that presented values in the range of 463 and 1444 ppm [46]. In addition, the highest content of α-tocopherol and total tocopherol was found in the yellow variety of Maranganí. Additionally, in Buenos Aires, four tocopherol vitamers were found, where y-tocopherol was the one with the highest content, followed by α-tocopherol, where its content was 0.9 and 3.1 mg [46]. Continuing, tocopherol investigations were also carried out in nine varieties of quinoa from four countries, counting Peru again, Bolivia, Colombia, and Denmark; the results showed two isoforms of tocotrienol and the β isoform of tocopherol were not present in the pigmented and non-pigmented varieties. Finally, Melini, V. & Melini, F mention that through all their research, α-, β-, γ-, and δ-tocopherol have been identified in 39 pigmented and non-pigmented quinoa samples, where γ- tocopherol was the most abundant, and the black genotypes were more abundant than the white varieties [46].

7.2.3 Phytoecdysteroids

They are a broad group of plant steroids where their structure is characterized by having a 5 β-cholestanol steroid skeleton that contains a 6-ketone ring B and a hydroxyl group at the C-14 α position. On the other hand, the study of phytoecdysteroids in quinoa and few investigations have been reported, such as the investigation of Chilean quinoa varieties and commercial samples of quinoa, where the total content of phytoecdysteroids was in the range of 224 and 570 $\mu g g^{-1}$ fw in Chilean samples, and in commercial samples it presented 138 and 568 $\mu g g^{-1}$ f [46].

Additionally, they were also carried out in 15 varieties of quinoa grains in Peru, department of Puno, for the content of phenolic compounds where they obtained a variation of 35.29–139.94 mg gallic acid per 100 grams [47] (**Table 7**).

In relation to other bioactive compounds in quinoa seed ecotypes, the content of deidzaine isoflavones was found in a range of 0.7–1.15 mg per 100 grams and 0.05–0.25 mg of genistein per 100 grams. On the other hand, a carotenoid content in the range of 1.69–3.88 mg per kilogram has also been recorded [48].

Flavonoids	Phenolic acids
Myricetin	Caffeic
Quercetin	Ferulic
Kaempferol	p-Hydroxybenzoic
Isohamnetin	Vanillinic
Routine	Gallic
Orientina	Cynamic
Vitexin	Protocatechuic
Morina	p-Cumaric
Hesperidin	—
Neohesperidin	—

Source: Taylor et al. (2014).

Table 7.
The flavonoids and phenolic acids identified in quinoa seeds.

8. Quinoa oil production methods

The process for the extraction of quinoa oil is described and is as follows [49]:

8.1 Receipt of the quinoa seed

The quinoa is received in bags of double Kraft paper material weighing 25 kg, later stored at room temperature and in a dry environment (**Figure 4**).

8.2 Cleaning

Cleaning is carried out manually in order to eliminate any impurities, such as defective seeds, stones, etc. (**Figure 5**).

8.3 Washed

Cold water was used for washing in order to eliminate the amount of saponin, which generates a detergency that is visualized by the creation of foam. At this stage, the seed has been polished, since the outer layer is removed (**Figure 6**).

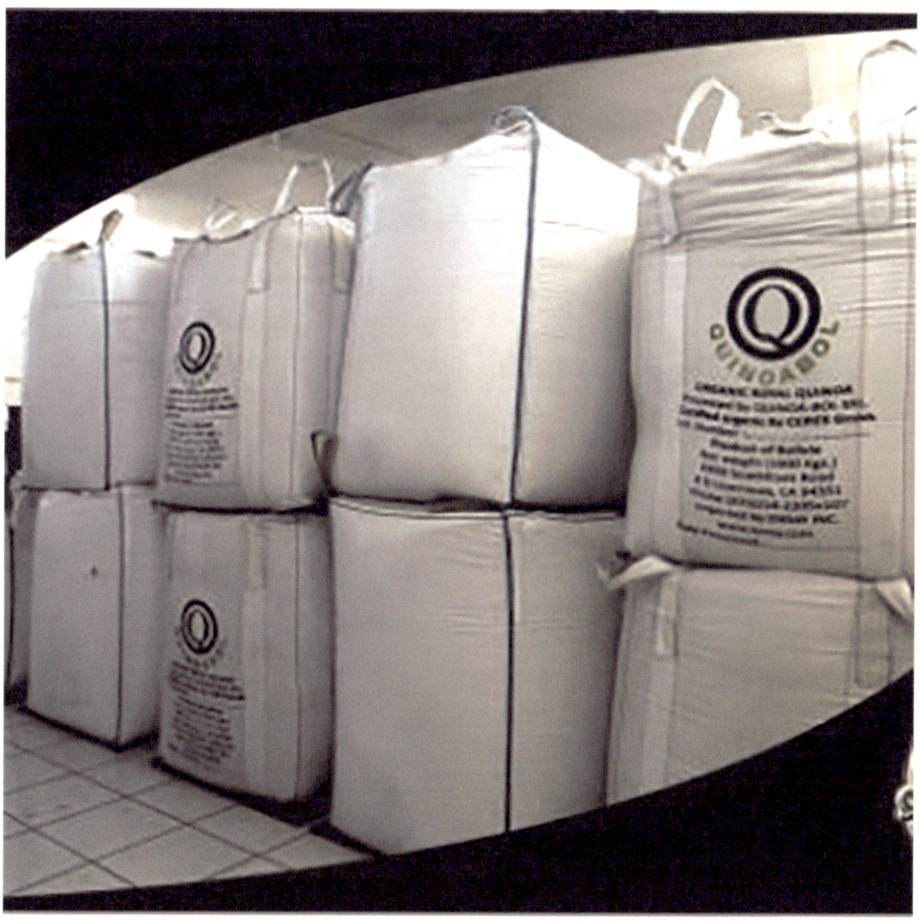

Figure 4.
25 kg bags of quinoa.

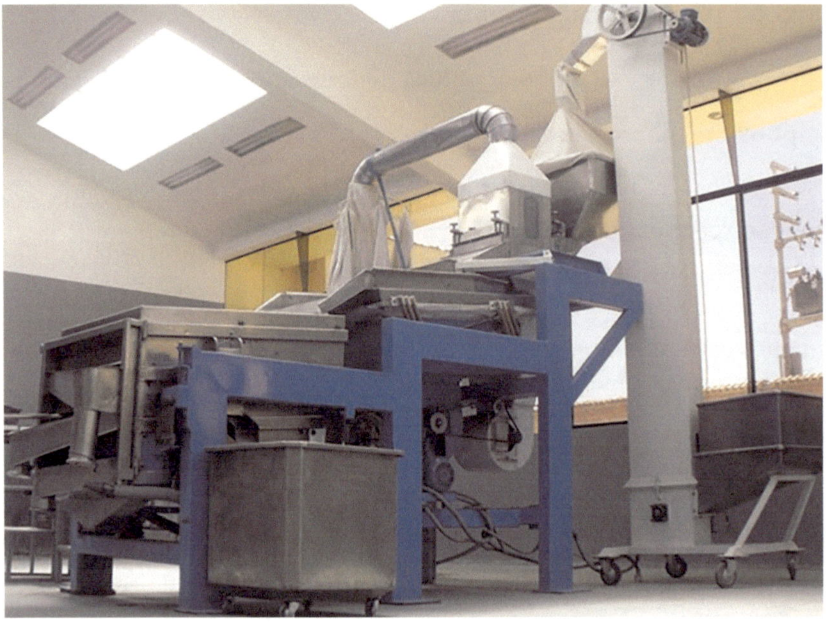

Figure 5.
Cleaning the quinoa grains.

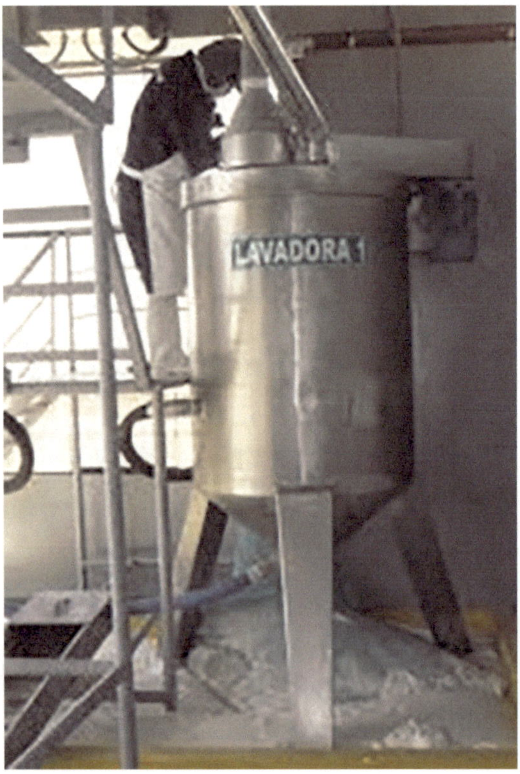

Figure 6.
Washing the quinoa.

8.4 Drying

The drying stage was carried out in a forced air oven at a temperature of 80° C with a time of 3 hours until a humidity of 8% is achieved (**Figure 7**).

8.5 Grinding

The milling was carried out with a hammer mill; this allows to reduce the size of the particles of the quinoa seeds, which allows us to break the cells, which makes the release of the oil feasible. In addition, the average size is 240 u of the particles (**Figure 8**).

8.6 Solvent extraction (hexane or petroleum ether)

The machine used to extract the oil was a Soxhlet extractor, which has a capacity of 3 kg. For this process, the already ground quinoa is placed in a basket in which it is in contact with the solvent. Finally, the duration of the process is observed until no more oil remains can be seen inside the machine (**Figure 9**).

8.7 Solvent evaporation

In this stage, the solvent is mixed with the quinoa oil; for this, it is evaporated in a rotary evaporator, where the solvent is divided with the oil (**Figure 10**).

8.8 Storage

Finally, the oil that is extracted and placed in glass bottles with an amber color and protected from light.

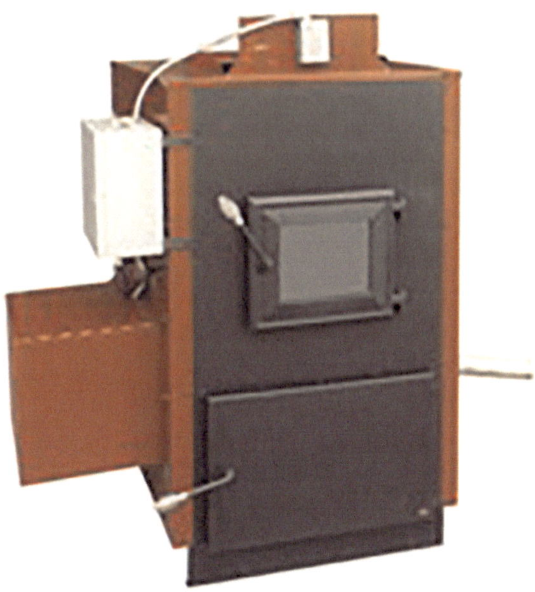

Figure 7.
Forced air stove.

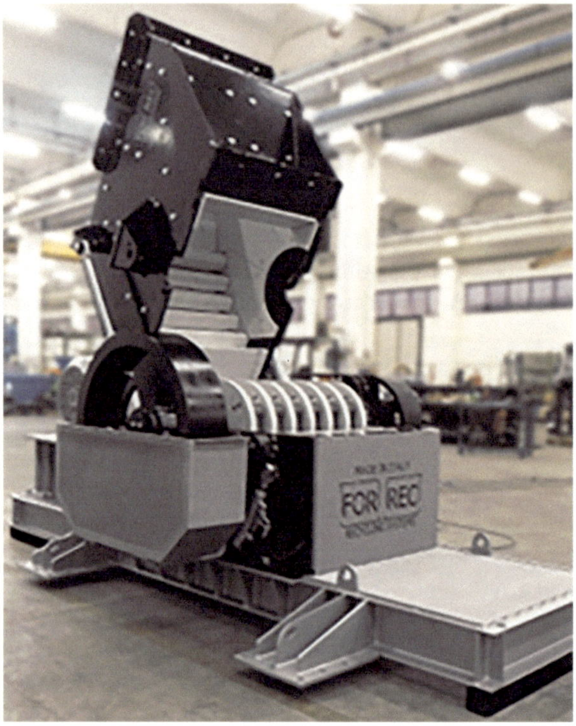

Figure 8.
Hammer mill.

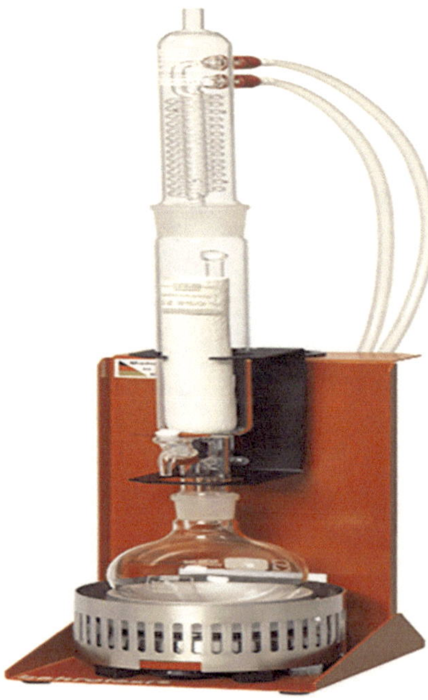

Figure 9.
Soxhlet extractor.

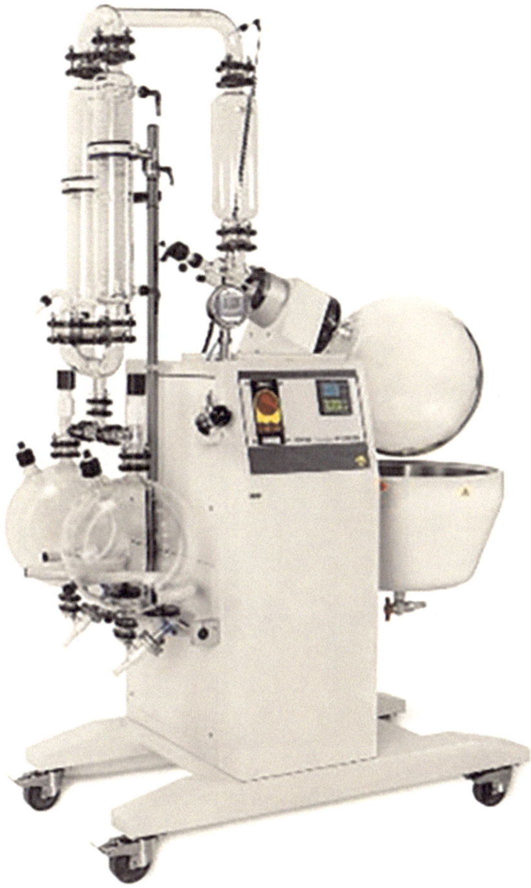

Figure 10.
Rotavapor.

9. Quinoa-based protein concentrate

The process of obtaining protein concentrate based on quinoa will be shown below [50]:

9.1 Sample preparation

The grain was cleaned and classified, subsequently a washing was carried out with distilled water and followed by drying at a temperature of 75°C for 8 hours. Furthermore, the saponin-free grains were ground, and a particle size of 25 μm was reached with a sieve.

9.2 Alkaline solubilization

A flour suspension was made, using distilled water with a 1:10 (w / v) ratio, and the pH is regulated with 1 N NaOH until reaching pH 9. Additionally, this suspension was moved for a time of 1 hour, the supernatant was taken (first extraction (and the precipitate was re-carried out in the solubilization process (second extraction).

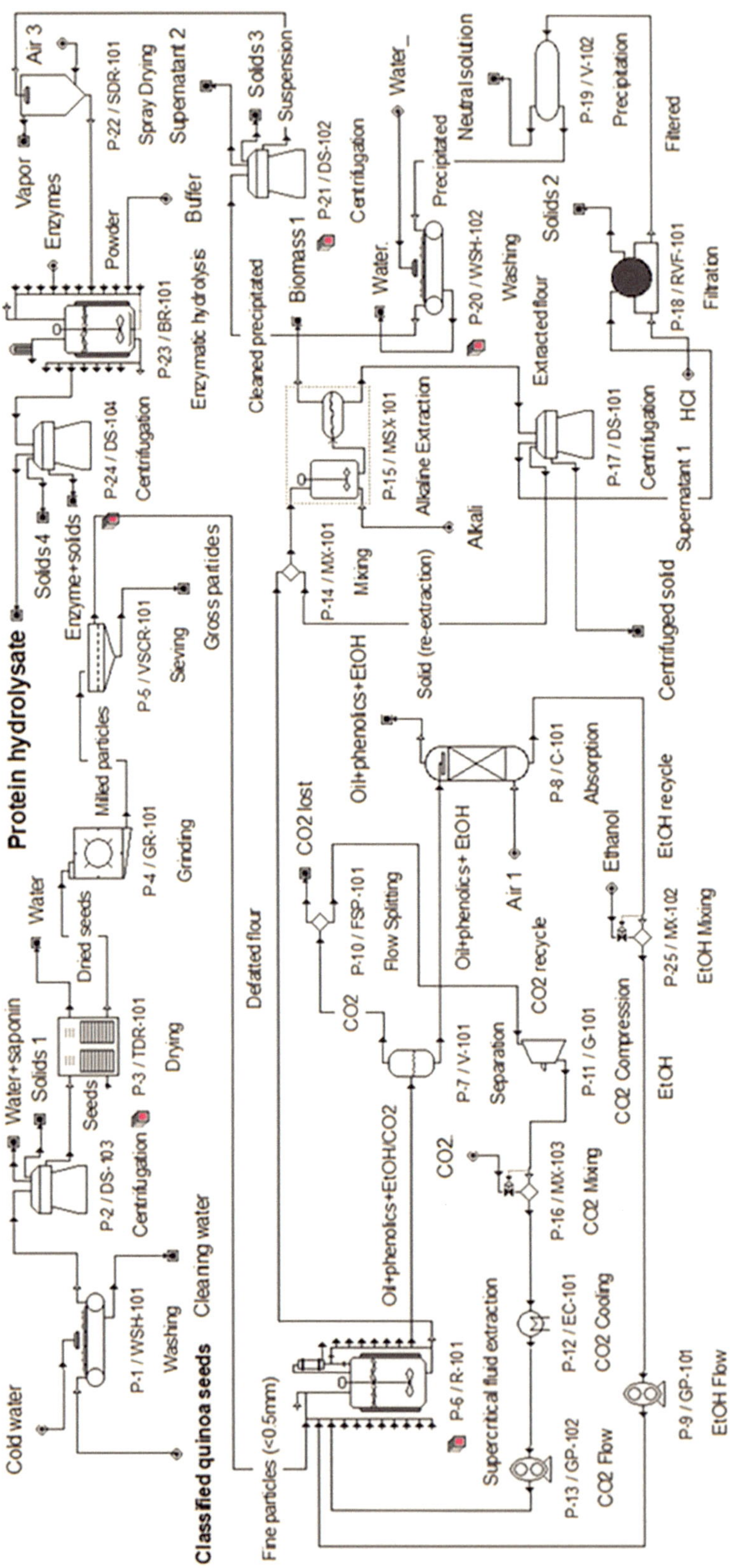
Protein hydrolysate
Cold water
Classified quinoa seeds
P-1 / WSH-101
Washing
Cleaning water
Water+saponin
Solids 1
P-2 / DS-103
Centrifugation
Seeds
P-3 / TDR-101
Drying
Water
Dried seeds
P-4 / GR-101
Grinding
Milled particles
P-5 / VSCR-101
Sieving
Gross particles
Enzyme+solids
Solids 4
P-24 / DS-104
Centrifugation
P-23 / BR-101
Enzymatic hydrolysis
Enzymes
Powder
Buffer
Vapor
Air 3
P-22 / SDR-101
Spray Drying
Supernatant 2
Solids 3
Suspension
P-21 / DS-102
Centrifugation
Cleaned precipitated
Biomass 1
Water.
Water_
Precipitated
P-20 / WSH-102
Washing
Neutral solution
P-19 / V-102
Precipitation
Filtered
Solids 2
P-18 / RVF-101
Filtration
Extracted flour
HCl
P-17 / DS-101
Centrifugation
Supernatant 1
Centrifuged solid
P-15 / MSX-101
Alkaline Extraction
Alkali
P-14 / MX-101
Mixing
Solid (re-extraction)
Oil+phenolics+EtOH
Defatted flour
Fine particles (<0.5mm)
P-6 / R-101
Supercritical fluid extraction
Oil+phenolics+EtOH/CO2
CO2 lost
P-10 / FSP-101
Flow Splitting
CO2
P-7 / V-101
Separation
Oil+phenolics+ EtOH
P-8 / C-101
Absorption
Air 1
CO2 recycle
P-11 / G-101
CO2 Compression
Ethanol
EtOH recycle
P-25 / MX-102
EtOH Mixing
EtOH
CO2
P-16 / MX-103
CO2 Mixing
P-12 / EC-101
CO2 Cooling
P-13 / GP-102
CO2 Flow
P-9 / GP-101
EtOH Flow

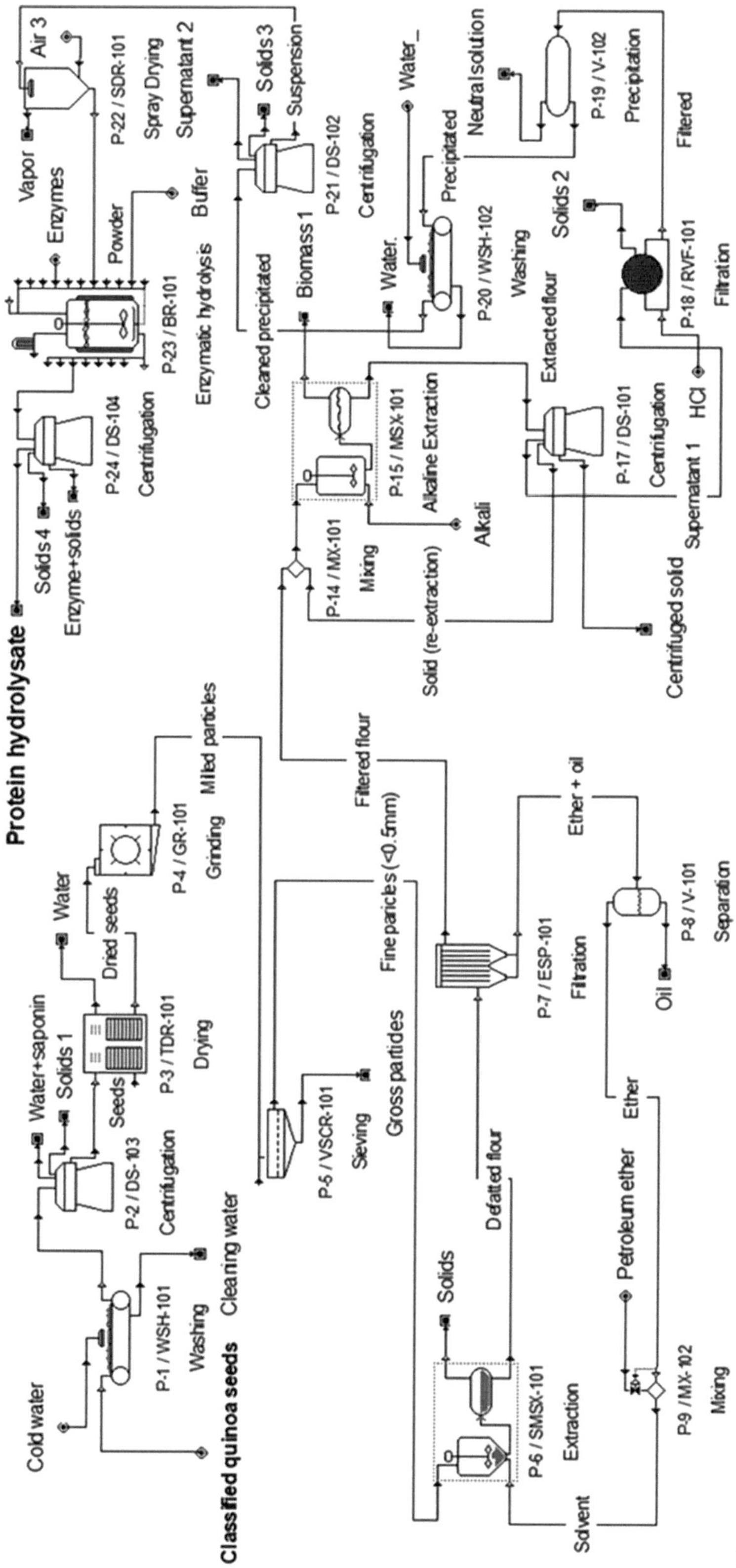

Figure 11.
Simulation flowsheet designed with SuperPro Designer 9® for the QPH production process using (a) SFE and (b) CSE.

9.3 Isoelectric precipitation

From the previous step, the collected supernatants, their pH were regulated with citric and hydrochloric acid until reaching a value of 4.5. The samples were centrifuged for a time of 15 minutes. Subsequently, the supernatant was discarded and with the precipitate, they were lyophilized at a temperature of −30°C. Finally, the samples obtained were placed in polyethylene material sleeves.

10. Economic evaluation at industrial scale of the production process of quinoa protein hydrolysates

A new method was proposed to obtain protein hydrolysates from quinoa, using supercritical fluids extraction (SFE), CO_2 and ethanol as cosolvent as a previous step to separate the fat and phenolic compounds in a single extraction process, and this was compared with the conventional solvent extraction (CSE) [51]. The production of quinoa protein hydrolysate (QPH) using two technologies to extract the oil and separate the phenolic compounds (PC) prior to enzymatic hydrolysis was evaluated: (1) Supercritical fluid extraction (SFE) and (2) Conventional solvent extraction (CSE). The aim of this study was to compare the oil extraction yield, remaining PC and QPH yield. Furthermore, an economic evaluation and sensitivity study was performed using SuperPro Designer 9.0 software; quinoa grain batches of 1.5 kg (laboratory) and 2500 kg (industrial scale) were considered, as shown in **Figure 4**. Results revealed that SFE allows higher oil yield and separation of PC. The cost of manufacturing (COM) was lower in SFE compared with CSE, US$ 90.10/kg and US$ 109.29/kg, respectively, and higher net present value (NPV), US$ 205,006,000 and US$ 28,159,000 compared with CSE. The best scenario is when the sale of both by-products (oil and saponins) is included, the COM is reduced to US$ 28.90/kg (SFE) and US$ 57.06/kg (CSE), and profitability also improves. In addition, the significance the COM and NPV was statistically evaluated, there are no significant differences on an industrial scale. Both processes are economically promising, especially when the QPH and by-products are produced in large scale and sold at the current market price (**Figure 11**).

11. Conclusions

Quinoa is a food that is produced mainly in Peru, Bolivia, and Ecuador and has nutritional characteristics superior to many vegetables. It is recognized as a complete food due to the quality of proteins, fiber, minerals, and vitamins; in addition to being gluten-free, it has allowed the development of new food products and is even used in an unconventional way as a nutraceutical, in the production of edible films, and as a stabilizing agent for emulsions.

However, quinoa grains have saponin, an anti-nutritional factor that can be eliminated by wet or dry methods, although there are some disadvantages such as high-water consumption, loss of essential nutrients such as vitamins, minerals, and amino acids, among others. It is therefore important to promote new methods of saponin elimination together with the development of breeding programs for quinoa varieties with low saponin content to improve yields per hectare.

The type of pretreatment with SFE and CSE applied to quinoa flour prior to enzymatic hydrolysis influences on the oil yield, remaining phenolic compounds and hydrolysate yield. The significance analysis of the factors considered shows that there is no significant effect on the COM and NPV of the QPH production at industrial scale between each technology; however, the pretreatment with SFE allows obtaining a lower COM and higher NPV, the sensitivity study and the evaluated scenarios show an additional income generated by the sale of by-products such as saponins and oils. Finally, it is corroborated by the values obtained, which as the scale of production increases, the manufacturing cost decreases for both technologies, making the production of quinoa protein hydrolysate viable at an industrial level.

Author details

Luis Olivera*, Ivan Best, Perla Paredes, Neyma Perez, Luis Chong and Alejandro Marzano
Food Science, Technology and Innovation Group, San Ignacio de Loyola University, Lima, Peru

*Address all correspondence to: lolivera@usil.edu.pe

References

[1] Ahumada A, Ortega A, Chito D, Benítez R. Saponinas de quinua (Chenopodium quinoa Willd.): Un subproducto con alto potencial biológico. Revista Colombiana de Ciencia Químico-Farmacéuticas. 2016;**45**(3):438-469. DOI: 10.15446/rcciquifa.v45n3.62043

[2] Jancurová M, Minarovičová L, Dandár A. Quinoa - A review. Czech Journal of Food Sciences. 2009;**27**(2): 71-79. DOI: 10.17221/32/2008-cjfs

[3] Kuljanabhagavad T, Wink M. Biological activities and chemistry of saponins from Chenopodium quinoa Willd. Phytochemistry Reviews. 2009; **8**(2):473-490. DOI: 10.1007/s11101-009-9121-0

[4] Bernal Mamani A, Padilla Hancco JA. Efecto de exopolisacáridos de lactobacillus reuteri en la elaboración de masa madre con harina de quinua (Chenopodium Quinoa Willd) variedad blanca "Salcedo Inia" y roja "Pasankalla". para la obtención de pan acido libre de gluten», *Univ. Nac. San Agustín Arequipa*. [En línea]. 2014. Disponible en: http://repositorio.unsa.edu.pe/handle/UNSA/4167 [Accedido: November 03, 2021].

[5] Repo-Carrasco-Valencia RA-M, Serna LA. Quinoa (Chenopodium quinoa, Willd.) as a source of dietary fiber and other functional components. Food Science and Technology. 2011;**31**: 225-230. DOI: 10.1590/S0101-20612011000100035

[6] Vilcacundo R, Hernández-Ledesma B. Nutritional and biological value of quinoa (Chenopodium quinoa Willd.). Current Opinion in Food Science. 2017;**14**:1-6. DOI: 10.1016/j.cofs.2016.11.007

[7] Huillca Huaman MH. Comparativo de rendimiento de grano, caracterización botánica, comportamiento fenológico y contenido de saponina de 11 líneas promisorias de quinua (Chenopodium quinoa Willdenow) bajo condiciones del Centro Agronómico K'ayra - Cusco», *Univ. Nac. San Antonio Abad Cusco*. [En línea]. 2019. Disponible en: http://repositorio.unsaac.edu.pe/handle/20.500.12918/3570 [Accedido: November 03, 2021]

[8] Hussain MI, Farooq M, Syed QA, Ishaq A, Al-Ghamdi AA, Hatamleh AA. Botany, nutritional value, phytochemical composition and biological activities of quinoa. Plants. 2021;**10**(11):2258. DOI: 10.3390/plants10112258

[9] FAO. Descriptors for quinoa and its wild relatives (In Spanish) - International Year of Quinoa. 2013. Disponible en: https://www.fao.org/quinoa-2013/publications/detail/en/item/201740/icode/?no_mobile=1 [Accedido: November 17, 2021]

[10] Christensen SA et al. Assessment of genetic diversity in the USDA and CIP-FAO international nursery collections of quinoa (Chenopodium quinoa Willd.) using microsatellite markers. Plant Genetic Resources. 2007; **5**(2):82-95. DOI: 10.1017/S1479262107672293

[11] Prego I, Maldonado S, Otegui M. Seed structure and localization of reserves in *Chenopodium quinoa*. Annals of Botany. 1998;**82**(4):481-488. DOI: 10.1006/anbo.1998.0704

[12] Scanlin L, Lewis KA. Quinoa as a sustainable protein source. In: Sustainable Protein Sources. London: Elsevier, Academic Press; 2017. pp. 223-238. DOI: 10.1016/B978-0-12-802778-3.00014-7

[13] Alandia G, Rodriguez JP, Jacobsen S-E, Bazile D, Condori B. Global expansion of quinoa and challenges for the Andean region. Global Food Security. 2020;**26**: 100429. DOI: 10.1016/j.gfs.2020.100429

[14] Abugoch James LE. Chapter 1 Quinoa (Chenopodium quinoa Willd.): Composition, chemistry, nutritional, and functional properties. In: Advances in Food and Nutrition Research. Vol. 58. Academic Press; 2009. pp. 1-31. DOI: 10.1016/S1043-4526(09)58001-1

[15] Wright KH, Pike OA, Fairbanks DJ, Huber CS. Composition of Atriplex hortensis, Sweet and Bitter Chenopodium quinoa Seeds. Journal of Food Science. 2002;**67**(4):1383-1385. DOI: 10.1111/j.1365-2621.2002.tb10294.x

[16] Bruin AD. Investigation of the food value of Quinua and Cañihua seed. Journal of Food Science. 1964;**29**(6): 872-876. DOI: 10.1111/j.1365-2621.1964.tb00464.x

[17] Lalaleo L, Hidalgo D, Valle M, Calero-Cáceres W, Lamuela-Raventós RM, Becerra-Martínez E. Differentiating, evaluating, and classifying three quinoa ecotypes by washing, cooking and germination treatments, using 1H NMR-based metabolomic approach. Food Chemistry. 2020;**331**:127351. DOI: 10.1016/j.food chem.2020.127351

[18] Mhada M, Metougui ML, El Hazzam K, El Kacimi K, Yasri A. Variations of saponins, minerals and total phenolic compounds due to processing and cooking of quinoa (Chenopodium quinoa Willd.) seeds. Food. 2020; **9**(5):660. DOI: 10.3390/foods905 0660

[19] Romano N, Ureta MM, Guerrero-Sánchez M, Gómez-Zavaglia A. Nutritional and technological properties of a quinoa (Chenopodium quinoa Willd.) spray-dried powdered extract. Food Research International. 2020;**129**: 108884. DOI: 10.1016/j.foodres.2019. 108884

[20] Kozioł MJ. Chemical composition and nutritional evaluation of quinoa (Chenopodium quinoa Willd.). Journal of Food Composition and Analysis. 1992; **5**(1):35-68. DOI: 10.1016/0889-1575(92) 90006-6

[21] Dini A, Rastrelli L, Saturnino P, Schettino O. A compositional study of Chenopodium quinoa seeds. Food / Nahrung. 1992;**36**(4):400-404. DOI: 10.1002/food.19920360412

[22] Repo-Carrasco R, Espinoza C, Jacobsen S-E. Nutritional value and use of the Andean crops Quinoa (Chenopodium quinoa) and Kañiwa (Chenopodium pallidicaule). Food Reviews International. 2003;**19**(1-2): 179-189. DOI: 10.1081/FRI-120018884

[23] Vega-Gálvez A, Miranda M, Vergara J, Uribe E, Puente L, Martínez EA. Nutrition facts and functional potential of quinoa (Chenopodium quinoa willd.), an ancient Andean grain: A review. Journal of the Science of Food and Agriculture. 2010;**90**(15):2541-2547. DOI: 10.1002/jsfa.4158

[24] Mohamed Ahmed IA, Al Juhaimi F, Özcan yMM. Insights into the nutritional value and bioactive properties of quinoa (Chenopodium quinoa): Past, present and future prospective. International Journal of Food Science and Technology. 2021;**56**(8):3726-3741. DOI: 10.1111/ijfs.15011

[25] Alvarez-Jubete L, Arendt EK, Gallagher E. Nutritive value and chemical composition of pseudocereals as gluten-free ingredients. International

Journal of Food Sciences and Nutrition. 2009;**60**(sup4):240-257. DOI: 10.1080/09637480902950597

[26] Ruales J, Nair BM. Saponins, phytic acid, tannins and protease inhibitors in quinoa (Chenopodium quinoa, Willd) seeds. Food Chemistry. 1993;**48**(2): 137-143. DOI: 10.1016/0308-8146(93)90048-K

[27] Valencia-Chamorro SA. QUINOA. In: Encyclopedia of Food Sciences and Nutrition. Amsterdam: Elsevier, Academic Press; 2003. pp. 4895-4902. DOI: 10.1016/B0-12-227055-X/00995-0

[28] Benito-Román O, Rodríguez-Perrino M, Sanz MT, Melgosa R, Beltrán S. Supercritical carbon dioxide extraction of quinoa oil: Study of the influence of process parameters on the extraction yield and oil quality. Journal of Supercritical Fluids. 2018;**139**:62-71. DOI: 10.1016/j.supflu.2018.05.009

[29] Graf BL, Rojas-Silva P, Rojo LE, Delatorre-Herrera J, Baldeón ME, Raskin I. Innovations in health value and functional food development of quinoa (*Chenopodium quinoa* Willd.). Comprehensive Reviews in Food Science and Food Safety. 2015;**14**(4):431-445. DOI: 10.1111/1541-4337.12135

[30] Ahamed NT, Singhal RS, Kulkarni PR, Pal M. Un grano menos conocido, Chenopodium Quinoa : Revisión de la composición química de sus partes comestibles. Food and Nutrition Bulletin. 1998;**19**(1):61-70. DOI: 10.1177/156482659801900110

[31] Elsohaimy SA, Refaay TM, Zaytoun MAM. Physicochemical and functional properties of quinoa protein isolate. Annals of Agricultural Science. 2015; **60**(2):297-305. DOI: 10.1016/j.aoas.2015.10.007

[32] Bhargava A, Shukla S, Ohri D. Chenopodium quinoa—An Indian perspective. Industrial Crops and Products. 2006;**23**(1):73-87. DOI: 10.1016/j.indcrop.2005.04.002

[33] Konishi Y, Hirano S, Tsuboi H, Wada M. Distribution of minerals in quinoa (Chenopodium quinoa Willd.) seeds. Bioscience, Biotechnology, and Biochemistry. 2004;**68**(1):231-234. DOI: 10.1271/bbb.68.231

[34] Talavera R. Determinación de la variedad de quinua expandida para elaboración de bombones», Universidad Nacional del Altiplano UNA-Puno, Ingeniería Agroindustrial, Puno. [En línea]. 2003. Disponible en: https://www.bioversityinternational.org/fileadmin/_migrated/uploads/tx_news/1411_Investigaciones_sobre_especies_olvidadas_y_subutilizadas_Granos_Andinos_Quinua_canahua_canihua_y_amaranto_kiwicha._Res%C3%BAmenes_de_trabajos_de_grado_y_tesis_de_maestr%C3%ADa_realizadas.pdf

[35] Srujana MNS, Kumari BA, Suneetha WJ, Prathyusha P. Processing technologies and health benefits of quinoa. The Pharma Innovation Journal. 2019;**8**(5):155-160

[36] Angeli V, et al. Quinoa (Chenopodium quinoa Willd.): An overview of the potentials of the "golden grain" and socio-economic and environmental aspects of its cultivation and marketization. Food. 2020;9(2):216. DOI: 10.3390/foods9020216

[37] Wang S, Zhu F. Formulation and quality attributes of quinoa food products. Food Bioprocessing Technology. 2016;**9**(1):49-68. DOI: 10.1007/s11947-015-1584-y

[38] El Hazzam K et al. An insight into saponins from quinoa (Chenopodium

quinoa Willd): A review. Molecules. 2020;**25**(5):1059. DOI: 10.3390/molecules25051059

[39] Heng L et al. Stability of pea DDMP saponin and the mechanism of its decomposition. Food Chemistry. 2006; **99**(2):326-334. DOI: 10.1016/j.foodchem.2005.07.045

[40] Hernández-Ledesma B. Quinoa (Chenopodium quinoa Willd.) as source of bioactive compounds: A review. Bioactive Compounds in Health and Disease. 2019;**2**(3):27-47. DOI: 10.31989/bchd.v2i3.556

[41] Madl T, Sterk H, Mittelbach M, Rechberger GN. Tandem mass spectrometric analysis of a complex triterpene saponin mixture of *Chenopodium quinoa*. Journal of the American Society for Mass Spectrometry. 2006;**17**(6):795-806. DOI: 10.1016/j.jasms.2006.02.013

[42] Jarvis DE et al. The genome of Chenopodium quinoa. Nature. 2017; **542**(7641):307-312. DOI: 10.1038/nature21370

[43] Sani Cujilema EJ. Obtención de emulsionantes a partir de saponina de Quinua (Chenopodium quinoa) por reacciones de esterificación para uso cosmético. [En línea]. 2019. Disponible en: http://dspace.espoch.edu.ec/handle/123456789/13955 [Accedido: November 05, 2021]

[44] Gunsha Allauca LJ. Elaboración de un emulsionante cosmético a base de las saponinas del agua de lavado de quinua (Chenopodium quinoa) en ERPE. [En línea]. 2013. Disponible en: http://dspace.espoch.edu.ec/handle/123456789/2471 [Accedido: November 05, 2021]

[45] Stuardo M, San Martín R. Antifungal properties of quinoa (Chenopodium quinoa Willd) alkali treated saponins against Botrytis cinerea. Industrial Crops and Products. 2008;**27**(3):296-302. DOI: 10.1016/j.indcrop.2007.11.003

[46] Melini V, Melini F. Functional components and anti-nutritional factors in gluten-free grains: A focus on quinoa seeds. Food. 2021;**10**:351. DOI: 10.3390/foods10020351

[47] Repo of Carrasco R, Encina-Zelada CR. Determination of the antioxidant capacity and phenolic compounds of Andean cereals: Quinoa (Chenopodium quinoa), kañiwa (Chenopodium pallidicaule) and kiwicha (Amaranthus caudatus). Magazine of the Chemical Society of Peru. 2008;**74**(2):85-99

[48] Lutz M, Martínez A, Martínez EA. Daidzein and genistein contents in seeds of quinoa (Chenopodium quinoa Willd.) From local ecotypes grown in arid Chile. Industrial Crops and Products. 2013;**49**: 117-121

[49] Rubio Y. QUINOA (Chenopodium qunoa Willd) OIL EXTRACTION AND ITS CHARACTERIZATION OF TWO ECOTYPES FROM THE COASTAL DRY OF REGION VI OF CHILE. University of Chile; 2005. Available from: http://www.hesis.uchile.cl/tesis/uchile/2005/rubio_y/sources/rubio_y.pdf

[50] Quelal M, Nazate K, Villacrés E, Cuarán J. Obtaining and characterizing a protein hydrolyzate of quinoa (Chenopodium quinoa Willd). Focus. 2019 Available from: https://www.redalyc.org/jatsRepo/5722/572262062007/html/index.html

[51] Olivera-Montenegro L, Best I, Gil-Saldarriaga A. Effect of pretreatment by supercritical fluids on antioxidant activity of protein hydrolyzate from quinoa (*Chenopodium quinoa* Willd.). Food Science & Nutrition. 2021;**9**(1): 574-582. DOI: 10.1002/fsn3.2027

Chapter 8

Metabolite Profile of *Amaranthus tricolor* L. and *Amaranthus cruentus* L. in Adaptation to Drought

Svetlana Motyleva, Murat Gins, Valentina Gins, Nikolay Tetyannikov, Ivan Kulikov, Ludmila Kabashnikova, Daria Panischeva, Maria Mertvischeva and Irina Domanskaya

Abstract

The Federal Research Center of Vegetable Growing has developed the cultivars Valentina (*Amaranthus tricolor* L.) and Krepysh (*Amaranthus cruentus* L.), which are successfully grown in several regions of Russia. The dry periods observed in recent years have a negative impact on the development of plants. The red-colored vegetable cultivar demonstrated a higher level of adaptability to drought than the green-colored grain cultivar. It was found that only in the leaves of cv. Valentina multiple spiked crystals consisting of four elements were formed, the predominant proportion belonged to Ca (38.59), then P (0.48), Mg (0.25), and K (0.16) followed, weight%, respectively. Under the conditions of moisture deficiency, the antioxidant activity of water and ethanol extracts in the leaves of both types of amaranth increased from 1.5 to 2.5 times. It was established that under drought conditions, the carbohydrate metabolism and the synthesis of secondary metabolites change. The leaves of the new cultivar of amaranth Valentina are a promising and reproducible source of antioxidants and can be used to create phytobiological preparations. The increased level of the main macro- and microelements—Ca, K, P, Mg, Mo, S and Cl in the seeds of cv. Valentina and Krepysh makes these cultivars promising for use in the food industry.

Keywords: amaranth, leaves, photosynthetic pigments, low-molecular-weight metabolites, ash composition of seeds

1. Introduction

Among abiotic stresses, drought is widely spread and strengthens from year to year all over the world. The stressful influence of drought conditions causes changes in morphological, physiological, and metabolical processes of plants that decrease the productivity and the quality of agricultural crops after all [1]. Molecular indicator of water stress is, first of all, speeded accumulation of active forms of oxygen that leads to the development of water stress, the change of chlorophylls structure, the decrease of photosynthetic pigments and metabolites, and the damage of plants cells [2–5].

Phenolic compounds and flavonoids are the most important and widely spread secondary products of plants. These metabolites enlarge enzymic antioxidant system and possess essential potential to decrease and prevent the cell damage [6]. Mineral elements are not only used as structural components, but also play an important role in the enzymes activity, osmotic pressure control for the cells' turgor and growth, take part in acid-base and water-salt metabolism [7–9]. Increased stability to drought mostly depends on the mineral composition of the plants [10, 11].

The most important and actual problem of genetic-breeding research studies is to determine the crops that are stable to drought. Metabolomic approach is a new direction of molecular-genetic research studies to identify the changes in plants under the influence of adverse environmental factors and to assess their nutritional value. Though, nowadays, the use of this approach remains a little used and poorly studied direction of breeding.

The fundamental knowledge about the characteristics of the leaves, seeds, and flour is crucial for the promotion of the crop for use in the food industry. The *Amaranthus tricolor* L.(cv. Valentina) leaf extracts do not only have beautiful crimson color, they also contain a large number of biologically active substances and can be used for tea drinks preparation. Amaranth gluten-free flour can be used for dietary bakery. This study is a first step toward a more efficient and successful application of amaranth as a commercially available pseudo-grain crop.

A. tricolor L. and *Amaranthus cruentus* L. species have been introduced and successfully grown in the Central region of Russia. However, during summer months, the dry period affects the productivity of these species negatively. Based on the foregoing, the present research work was also planned to evaluate and study the mechanisms of drought resistance of two species of amaranth under the conditions of artificial abiotic stress caused by drought.

2. Studies results

2.1 Studies place, objects, and methods

A vegetative experiment was conducted with amaranth species *A. tricolor* L. cv. Valentina (vegetable, red-colored cultivar, with the leaves and seeds having nutritional value for human organisms) and *A. cruentus* L. cv. Krepysh (grain, green-colored cultivar with the seeds having nutritional value for human organisms) in 2020–2021 in the department of gene pool and plant bioresources of the Federal Horticultural Research Center for Breeding, Agrotechnology and Nursery (FHRCBAN), Moscow. The plants of both species were placed outdoors with artificial protection from precipitation. The climate of the study site is moderately continental, the height above sea level is 168 m, the coordinates are 55° 7′27″ north latitude, 37° 56′ 55″. The amaranth plants were grown by seedlings and transplanted into plastic pots (250 and 175 mm in diameter and height, respectively) one plant per a pot. Totally 40 pots were planted, 20 pieces of each species: 10 control plants and 10 drought-affected ones.

The pots were filled with a mixture of peat and sand (5:1) with a drainage layer at the bottom. In the pots with the control samples, the humidity of the substrate for the plants was maintained at the level of 45–50%. Soil moisture was determined using soil moisture meter MC-7828 SOIL. All the plants were grown for 2 months in well-watered conditions in natural light (**Figure 1**). The average day/night temperature,

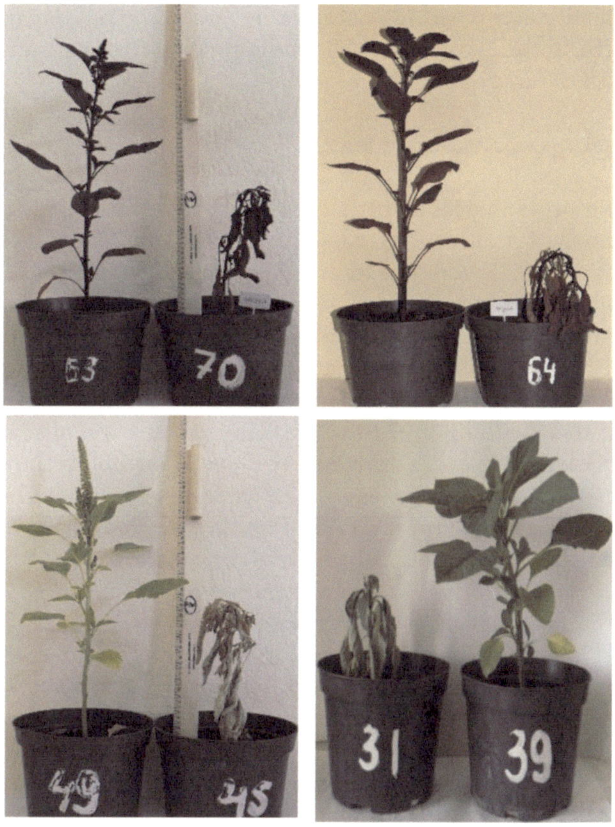

Figure 1.
General view of control plants A. tricolor *L. cv. Valentina and* A. cruentus *L. cv. Krepysh and drought-prone plants.*

relative humidity, and the day length during the experimental period were 17.2°C/ 11.7°C, 64%, and 17 h, respectively. After 2 months of growth, the degree of stress from drought was determined according to the moisture content in the soil. The watering of the experimental plants was stopped until the signs of wilting. The duration of the soil drought period was 7 days. The plants were examined when the soil moisture dropped till 20–25%.

The biochemical research studies were held in the Laboratory of Physiology and Biochemistry of FHRCBAN.

The understudied parameters included the laboratory studies of the leaves (microscopy of cross sections of the leaf blade, photosynthetic pigments content, antioxidant activity, phenolic compounds sum, ash composition seeds, and quality content of the leaves' main metabolites). The leaves' microscopy and ash composition were determined on analytical REM JEOL JSM-6010 LA (JEOL Ltd., Japan). Photosynthetic pigments Chl a and b and total carotenoids (Car) were studied on spectrophotometer Helios ϒ UV–vis (USA) in accordance with the method [12]. Total phenolic amount was determined with Folin–Ciocalteu reagent in accordance with the method [13] and total antioxidant capacity, the scavenging activity for the 2, 2-dipheny l-1-picrylhydrazyl (DPPH) radical was determined in accordance with the method [14].

Metabolites quality composition contained in leaf extracts was analyzed on JEOL JMS-Q1050GC (JEOL Ltd., Japan) via the method of gas chromate-mass-spectrometry in accordance with the method [15].

2.2 Biomineralization of amaranth leaves

An important morphological feature of *A. tricolor* L. cv. Valentina is biomineralization—the presence of multiple crystals in the leaf tissue. In the leaves of *A. cruentus* L. cv. Krepysh, the crystals were not found. The round spiked crystals (metabolic products) are often located on the transverse sections of the leaf of *A. tricolor* L. cv. Valentina between the adaxial and abaxial sides (**Figure 2**).

The local energy dispersive spectrometry (EDS) analysis showed that the inclusions contained four elements. The main element was Ca (5.9–8.3 mass %); K (0.34–0.38 mass%); Mg and P—0.03–0.07 mass %. The combination of scanning electron microscopy (SEM) and EDS was a convenient method for determining the microstructure in the cross section of the leaves of *Amarantus* L. X-rays showing the location of all the elements are presented in **Figure 3**. K, P, and Mg are evenly distributed around the mineral inclusions. Ca is concentrated in the crystal. The SEM/EDX results allowed determining the concentration and distribution of elements in the mineral inclusions in the leaves of *A. tricolor* L. cv. Valentina. Calcium oxalate (Ca) crystals are found in many plant species and in most organs and tissues of photosynthetic organisms [16–19]. The modern research studies say that Ca2+ is a key element of signaling pathways and is mobilized during the adaptation process to biotic and abiotic stresses [20–22].

Calcium is involved in regulating metabolic processes, plant growth and development [23]. Under drought stress, Ca is an integral part of the recovery process after stress exposure, regulating the plasma membrane enzyme adenosinetriphosphatase, which is required to pump back nutrients lost during cell damage [24].

2.3 Effects of drought on influence on photosynthetic pigments synthesis

The content analysis of chlorophylls and carotenoids in the amaranth leaves showed that some changes were associated with drought (**Figure 4**). An increase of Chl a, b and Car was observed in the leaves of drought-affected amaranth species. In the leaves of *A. tricolor* L. cv. Valentina, the content of Chl a doubled; on the other hand, a slight decrease in the content of Chl b was noted. In the leaves of *A. cruentus* L. cv. Krepysh, the content of Chl b increased slightly in comparison with the content of Chl a. The content of carotenoids in the amaranth leaves increased in the conditions of

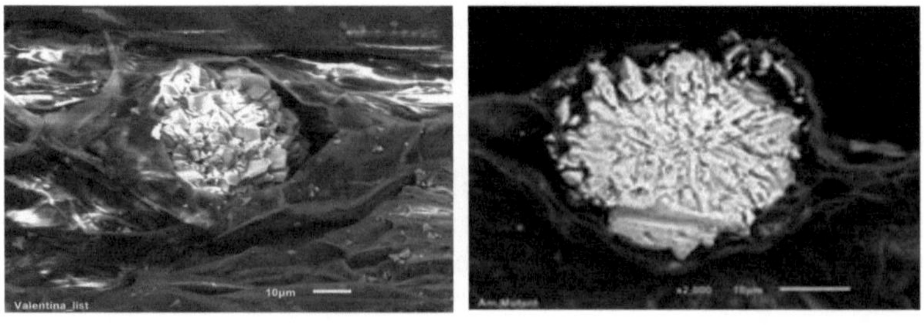

Figure 2.
The protrusions of crystals (a) and Mineral inclusions in the cross-section leaves Amaranthus tricolor *cv. Valentina.*

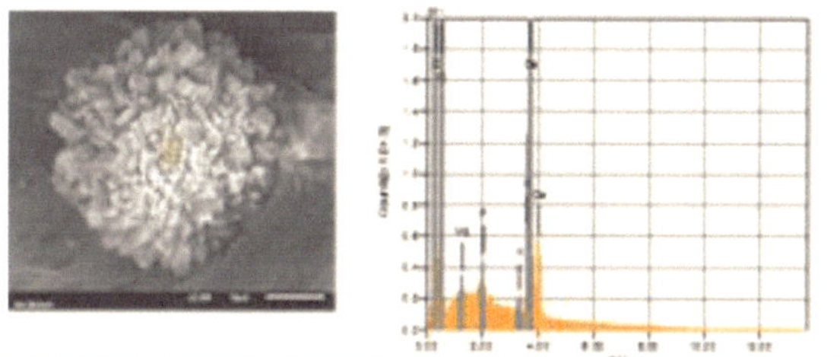

Minerals	Element content, wt %	Variation coefficient, (%)
Mg	0.25	0.74
P	0.48	0.47
Ca	38.59	0.09
K	0.16	0.38

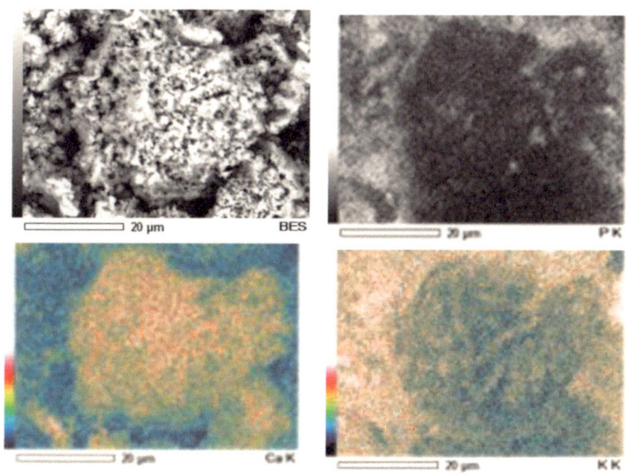

Figure 3.
Mineral inclusions in the cross section of amaranth leaves and EDS crystal alalysis. SEM micrographs and corresponding EDX spectra of elements in the cross-section leaves Amaranthus tricolor *cv. Valentina., sample 2000 X. The energy spectrum of the X-rays character emitted from the element of K, P and Ca.*

moisture deficiency: in the leaves of *A. tricolor* L., it increased 2.5 times, and in the leaves of *A. cruentus* L.—1.5–2.0 times compared with the control. These results are consistent with the data received from the testing on Choy sum in the dry season [25], which reported an increase in total carotenoid content under drought stress.

A high correlation was found between Chl a and Car (r = 0.985) and Chl b and Car (r = 0.977) in the leaves of *A. tricolor* L. and *A. cruentus* L., respectively. The observed changes in photosynthetic pigments of the leaves in drought are probably associated with free-radical-induced oxidation of Chl pigment [26], the destruction of some chloroplasts, and an increase in the activity of Chl catabolizing enzyme of chlorophyllase [27]. The increase in chlorophyll concentration under drought stress can be determined as an indicator of the plant tissues' resistance to abiotic stress under the drought conditions, which is fully consistent with the data of Jain et al., [28], who reported similar observations. Carotenoids are involved in drought stress resistance due to their ability to capture singlet oxygen. They can also inhibit lipid peroxidation

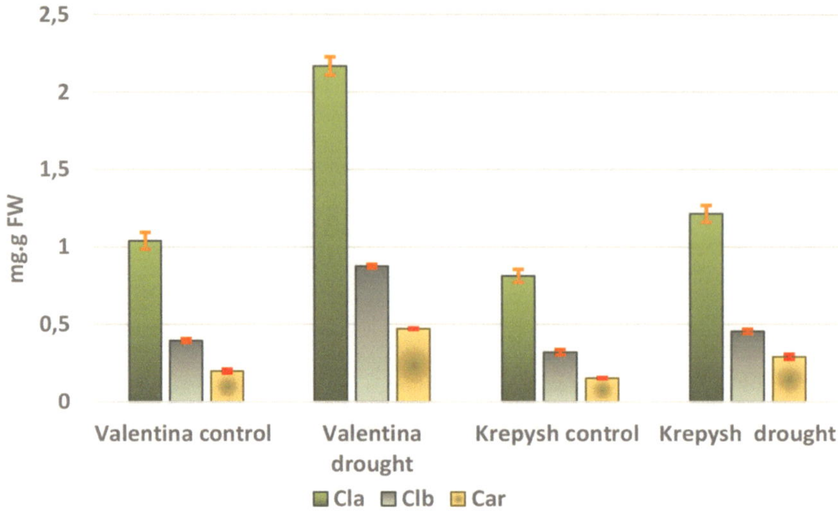

Figure 4.
The content of chlorophyll a *(Cla), chlorophyll* b *(Clb) and carotenoids (Car) in the leaves of amaranth (C4) under stress conditions of drought. Data are the mean ± SE of three replicates.*

and superoxide formation by dehydrating factors. Carotenoids and beta-carotene may play the main protective role in photosynthetic tissue as they directly help plants resist drought [29].

2.4 Effects of drought on influence on antioxidant activity and phenol compounds sum accumulation

The ability of amaranth leaf extracts to absorb DPPH + free radicals, which is used as a measure of total antioxidant activity (TAA), and total phenol content (TPC) are shown in **Table 1**. The antioxidant activity of the water extracts of *A. tricolor* L. leaves was significantly higher than that of *A. cruentus* L. leaves. The antioxidant activity of the alcohol solution differed slightly between the types of amaranth. In the conditions

Samples	Determined indicators		
	AAA	AAM	TPS
A. tricolor L., control V %	24.11 ± 1.87 7.75	16.26 ± 0.65 0.43	2.28 ± 0.37 16.06
A. tricolor L. drought V %	66.82 ± 1.36 2.03	27.08 ± 0.87 3.24	6.61 ± 0.56 8.59
A. cruentus L. control V %	1.35 ± 0.21 14.93	16.08 ± 0.24 1.53	1.15 ± 0.07 6.09
A. cruentus L. drought V %	7.71 ± 1.01 13.56	26.05 ± 0.56 2.15	3.19 ± 0.45 14.18

Table 1.
The effect of drought stress on the antioxidant activity of water (AAA) and methanol (AAM) extracts, expressed in %, and the total content of polyphenols (TPC), expressed in mg equivalent of gallic acid (mg/g TW) in the leaves of Amaranthus species.

of water deficiency in the leaves of both types of amaranth, the antioxidant activity of water and alcohol extracts increases by 1.5–2.5 times. Antioxidant activity plays a crucial role in maintaining the balance between free radical synthesis and capture [30–32]. With a lack of water, the total content of phenols in the leaves of both types of amaranth increases by three times. The variation coefficient of the antioxidant activity and the total amount of phenolic compounds was low, which indicates the relative homogeneity of the data obtained. A high correlation was established between the antioxidant activity of water and alcohol extracts and the TPC content in the leaves of both amaranth species (r = 0.77, r = 0.91), respectively.

Hence, the leaf mass of *A. tricolor* L. can be considered as a source of plant antioxidants that can normalize the ability of the human body to counteract free radicals caused by stress.

2.5 The influence of drought on the contents of metabolites in the leaves of A. tricolor L. (cv. Valentina) и A. cruentus L. (cv. Krepysh)

Forty-three secondary metabolites were totally determined in ethanol extracts of amaranth leaves. Forty-two substances were identified in the leaves of *A. tricolor* L. (cv. Valentina) and 35 metabolites in the leaves of *A. cruentus* L. (cv. Krepysh) (**Table 2**). Among nine compounds that possess antimicrobial characteristics, five belong to organic acids—Lactic acid, Pyruvic acid, Glyoxylic acid, Acetamide, Malic acid, and Tartaric acid; one to sugar alcohol—Glycerol; one to amide—Acetamide; and one to phenolic compounds—Benzoic acid. The content of Lactic acid, Benzoic acid, Malic acid, and Mannonic acid is 40, 6, 2, and 1.5 times higher in the leaves of cv. Valentina, than in the leaves of cv. Krepysh, respectively. Glyoxylic acid is found only in the leaves of green-colored amaranth; Acetamide is only in the leaves of red amaranth. Other organic acids are represented by the following compounds: Butanoic scid, Clycolic acid, Oxalic acid, 2-Butanedioic acid, Monoethyl malonic acid, Succinic acid, Glyceric acid, 2-Oxopentanoic acid, Malonic acid, 2.3.4.-Trihydroxybutiric acid, Arabinoic acid, Ketosuccinic acid, Fumaric acid, 2-Propenoic acid, and Citric acid. The phenolic compounds are presented by Caffeic acid, Vanillic acid, and Cinnamic acid. The following compounds were also detected: glycoside Apigenin, keto-acid—1.2-Ketoglutaric acid, sugar acid—Myo-inositol; 4 aminoacids—Lauric acid, Myristic acid, Palmitic acid, and Stearic acid (only in the leaves of cv. Valentina). Under drought conditions, the following compounds were synthesized in a significantly larger amount in the leaves of A. tricolor L. cv. Valentina: Mannonic acid—by 70 times; Myo-inositol—by 40 times; Caffeic acid—by 23 times; Tartaric acid—by 15 times; Clycerol—by 7 times; L-Proline and Serine—by 4 times; and Glycolic acid, Oxalic acid, and Lactic acid—by 2–3 times. The differences in the synthesis of these compounds were less obvious in the leaves of *A. cruentus* L. (cv. Krepysh). Our results are consistent with earlier findings that the accumulation of Proline and other amino acids increases with water potential decrease in the leaves [33, 34]. Myo-inositol is necessary for absolutely everyone for the synthesis of the substances involved in the transmission of intracellular signals from receptors. It is a vitamin-like substance that affects metabolism and normalizes the levels of sugar and insulin in the blood. It increases the sensitivity of body cells to hormones, supports hormonal balance, and stimulates the proper functioning of the hormone insulin and the stabilization of carbohydrate metabolism [35]. The present study confirmed that the leaves of cv. Valentina and Krepysh are the sources of biologically active compounds and have an enriched antioxidant profile.

N	Tmin	Metabolite	Peak height, % of scale cv. Valentina cv,Krepysh		Biological characteristic
1	**10:20**	**Lactic acid**	**15–8**	**0.3–0.2**	**Antimicrobial 93**
2	10:23	Butanoic scid	1.4–0.5	1.2–0.3	Organic acid
3	10:27	Clycolic acid	5–15	5–7	Organic acid
4	10:28	Oxalic acid	10–15	8–5	Organic acid
5	10:42	Pyruvic acid	0.2–0.2	0.3–1.2	Antimicrobial 118
6	10:49	2-Butanedioic acid	0.2–1.5	0.1–7	Organic acid
7	11:00	L-Alanine	1.5–4	1.2–1.8	Amino acid
8	11:29	Monoethyl malonic acid	8–10	5–10	Organic acid
9	12:16	Glyoxylic acid	—	2.5–3	Antimicrobial 78
10	13:23	Acetamide	0.8–0	—	Antimicrobial 40
11	13:43	Glycerol	8–60	8–70	Antimicrobial 77
12	14.04	Succinic acid	11–15	3–4	Organic acid
13	14:23	Glyceric acid	40–13	13–7	Organic acid
14	15:03	Glycine	0.4–3	0.2–1.5	Amino acid
15	15:24	2-Oxopentanoic acid	2–3.2	8–10	Organic acid
16	15:29	Malonic acid	6–7	2–3	Organic acid
17	16:27	Malic acid	14–27	8–19	Antimicrobial 96
18	16:40	L-5-Oxoproline	1.5–2	1.2–2	Amino acid derivative
19	16:48	L-Proline	5–20	4–11	Amino acid
20	17:30	2.3.4.-Trihydroxybutiric acid	22–43	—	Organic acid
21	17:54	1. 2-Ketoglutaric acid	0.2–0.4	—	Keto acid
22	18:14	Arabinoic acid	0.3–0.25	0.3–0.3	Organic acid
23	18:16	Ketosuccinic acid	11–8	—	Organic acid
24	18.24	Lauric acid	0.2–0.4	0.1	Saturated fatty acid
25	19:33	Vanillic acid	2–2.5	—	Phenolic acid
26	19:37	Benzoic acid	3–4.1	0.5–1.6	Antimicrobial 60
27	16.46	Fumaric acid	0.1–0.5	—	Organic acid
28	16:58	Serine	2.5–11	3–8	Amino acid
29	25:00	2-Propenoic acid	0.1–0.3	—	Organic acid
30	20:08	Adenine	1–4	1–2.5	Amino acid
31	20:21	Citric acid	15–40	8–15	Organic acid
32	21:48	Cinnamic acid	2.5–2.8	1.2–1.0	Phenolic acid
33	22:24	Myristic acid	4–13	4–10	Saturated fatty acid
34	22:26	Acrylic acid	8–10	6–10	Antimicrobial 44
35	22:30	Palmitic Acid	0.1	0.05–0.1	Saturated fatty acid
36	22:46	Tartaric acid	4–62	3–15	Antimicrobial 126
37	22:48	Caffeic acid	1.2–28	0.2–0.8	Phenolic acid

N	Tmin	Metabolite	Peak height, % of scale cv. Valentina cv,Krepysh		Biological characteristic
1	**10:20**	**Lactic acid**	**15–8**	**0.3–0.2**	**Antimicrobial 93**
38	23:17	Apigenin	0.4–1.2	—	Glycosides
39	23:31	Myo-inositol	10–40	11–15	Sucar acid
40	24:19	Stearic acid	1–1.4	—	Saturated fatty acid
41	34:14	Mannonic acid	10–70	8–30	Organic acid

Table 2.
Metabolites discovered in ethanol extracts of Amaranthus *L. leaves.*

2.6 The ash residue comparative composition of *A. tricolor* L. (Valentina cultivar) and *A. cruentus* L. (Krepysh cultivar) amaranth seeds

The content (in mass %) of 11 main elements that make up the mineral part of amaranth seeds was studied (**Table 3**). The ash composition of the seeds varies significantly. The descending series of the elements accumulation is the following:

A. tricolor L. – Ca > P > K > Mg > Mo > S > Si > Se > Fe > Zn > Mn.

A. cruentus L. – K > P > Ca > Mg > Mo > S > Se > Zn > Fe > Si > Mn.

At the same time, the main proportion of ash elements in the seeds of *A. tricolor* L. is Ca, and in the seeds of *A. cruentus* L.—K.

Ca is the main ash element in the seeds of *A. tricolor* L., and its portion is 17.83 mass %. The proportion of Ca in the seeds of *A. cruentus* L. is less, and its portion is 11.54 mass %. Ca is a part of coenzymes and cell nuclei, it is involved in the most important processes for human organisms, such as metabolism, immunity, regeneration, and others [36]. The proportion of K in the seeds of *A. cruentus* L. is 1.8, and the proportion

Mineral Elements	*Amaranthus tricolor* L. cv. Valentina			*Amaranthus cruentus* L. cv. Krepysh		
	$\bar{x}$. ±Sx	min-max	V,%	$\bar{x}$. ±Sx	min-max	V,%
K	8.94 ± 0.20	7.78–9.07	13.35	15.78 ± 0.19	11.71–13.32	17.75
P	9.67 ± 0.08	8.49–9.98	8.82	14.38 ± 0.15	13.29–14.87	27.78
Ca	17.83 ± 0.08	16.71–18.08	13.39	11.54 ± 0.12	9.76–14.37	29.85
Mo	2.54 ± 0.04	2.12–3.35	17.62	3.43 ± 0.04	3.21–4.86	45.16
Mg	7.33 ± 0.42	6.31–8.89	13.09	5.76 ± 0.22	4.06–6.06	38.21
S	1.84 ± 0.20	1.08–2.35	19.45	2.23 ± 1.04	1.49–2.41	38.60
Si	0.48 ± 0.07	0.41–0.64	20.68	0.21 ± 0.08	0.17–0.37	22.97
Mn	0.17 ± 0.11	0.12–0.21	27.81	0.19 ± 0.08	0.10–0.29	54.20
Fe	0.23 ± 0.04	0.18–0.36	36.38	0.23 ± 0.03	0.13–0.39	58.40
Zn	0.21 ± 0.06	0.17–0.34	30.35	0.26 ± 0.08	0.17–0.24	29.45
Se	0.41 ± 0.06	0.37–0.54	29.45	0.35 ± 0.06	0.27–0.44	31.18
∑	49.65			54,36		

*Notice: *significant at P < 0.05.*

Table 3.
Mineral (ash) composition of Amaranthus *L. seeds, mass %, X (2020–2021).*

of P is 1.5 times higher than that in the seeds of *A. tricolor* L. The macroelement K is responsible for regulating the majority of metabolic reactions occurring in living organisms. It controls osmotic pressure, transmembrane potential, charge equilibrium, cathode-anion balance, pH—everything that makes up the homeostasis of cells and tissues [37]. In the human body, P is a part of DNA and RNA, phospholipids, phosphate esters, nucleoside phosphates—ATP, ADP, NATP, where it performs a structural and metabolic function [38].

The content of Mg and Mo in the seeds of *A. tricolor* L. (7.33 and 2.54 mass %) differs slightly from the content in the seeds of *A. cruentus* L. (5.76 and 3.43 mass %). In the human body, Mg is necessary for the processes of regeneration and renewal of cells, tissues, and organs. It activates a large number of enzymes involved in the assimilation of CO_2 and nitrogen. In cytosol, Mg balances organic compounds (groups of sugars, nucleotides, organic and amino acids). Mg is necessary to maintain cathodic-anionic balance and regulate pH [39]. Mo is an important element in the diet, catalyzes the reactions of oxygen transfer from substrates or to substrates, using water as a donor or acceptor of oxygen, is a part of enzymes [40]. The content of trace elements S, Mn, Fe, and Zn in amaranth seeds of the studied cultivars differs slightly (**Table 2**).

S is a biogenic element in the composition of proteins and glutathione, has antioxidant activity, provides the process of energy transfer in the cell by transferring electrons, participates in the transfer and fixation of methyl groups, the formation of covalent, hydrogen, and mercaptide bonds, provides the transfer of genetic information. Mn is a cofactor and activator of many enzymes (pyruvate kinase, decarboxylase, siperoxide dismutase), participates in the synthesis of glycoproteins and proteoglycans, has antioxidant activity.

In active centers (hemoproteins and iron-sulfur proteins), Fe determines the structure and activity of space and participates in redox reactions. Organic Fe is a necessary compound for the human body. This element is part of catalytic centers of many redox enzymes. Zn stabilizes the structure of molecules, plays an important role in the metabolism of DNA and RNA, in protein synthesis and cell division, in the processes of signaling within the cell [41–43].

Si is not only the basis of the framework element of tissues, but also controls a number of biological and chemical processes in a living organism, increases the resistance of a living organism to the effects of biogenic and abiogenic stressors, is a necessary trace element that is part of active centers in the form of selenocysteine animoacystide [44]. The concentration of Si in *A. tricolor* L. seeds is two times more than that in the seeds of *A. cruentus* L.

The minerals found in amaranth seeds are important for meeting human dietary needs and can make a significant contribution to recommended diets.

2.7 Biologically active components of the studied cultivars of *Amaranthus L.*

The previous studies of the extracts from cv. Valentina fresh leaves detected the following physiologically active substances with antioxidant activity: Amarantin—1.5 mg/g, Ascorbic acid—150–170 mg/100 g, simple phenols and phenolcarboxylic acids, Chlorogenic, Ferulic, Gallic acids, and Arbutin—2.05, 0.01, 1.51, and 473 mg/g, respectively. All metabolites are biologically active substances [45]. Phenolic acids and Betacyanin (Amarantin) are characterized by antibacterial [46–48], antimycotic, anti-inflammatory, and wound-healing properties. Ferulic acid has radioprotective properties, glycosylated hydroquinone Arbutin exhibits antioxidant activity [48]. The pigment Amarantin is a multifunctional pigment of red-colored amaranth leaves. Amarantin is a nitrogenous heterocyclic compound that has a strong physiological effect on living organisms. The study of the biochemical properties of Amarantin extracted from the leaves of the red-colored cv. Valentina revealed the following physiological activities: antibacterial, antimycotic, antioxidant, antitumor. The extracts from fresh and dried leaves of cv. Valentina stimulated the growing activity of vegetable seeds, which allows its extracts to be used in phytobiology for stimulation of seeds and sprouts (in the concentration of 10-4, 10-5 M) [49]. The mechanism of antioxidant activity of Amarantin is associated with its ability to neutralize the superoxide radical and inhibit lipid peroxidation. This allows the leaves to be used to obtain Amarantin extract as a dietary supplement and a phytopreparation.

Under the conditions of drought and high solar radiation, the content of Amarantin in the leaves of cv. Valentina decreases to 40%. The received data indicate that Amarantin performs an important protective function of the photosynthetic apparatus in the plant [50, 51]. The advantage of Amarantin as a water-soluble antioxidant is its rapid synthesis (within 4 hours) after the cessation of drought. The data obtained by us and investigated in the literature data indicate an important role of Amarantin in photosynthetic, metabolic, and protective reactions of an amaranth plant.

Consequently, the data found in literary sources and the results received by us prove that *A. tricolor* L. cv. Valentina is not only highly drought-tolerant, but is also a promising, reproducible source of antioxidants and can be used to create functional foods and phytobiological preparations. The presence of potential antinutrients may limit the use of amaranth in a human diet. To inactivate or reduce these antinutrients, various pretreatment methods are used, such as heat treatment, extrusion, etc. Therefore, further profiling of the metabolomic profile is necessary to improve the nutritional properties of the food product.

3. Conclusions

In the present study, the representatives of species C4 (amaranth) *A. tricolor* L. cv. Valentina and *A. cruentus* L. cv. Krepysh have observed several adaptive responses to drought stress under the conditions of water deficit. The features of specific changes in photosynthetic pigments, antioxidant activity, the amount of phenolic compounds, and the composition of metabolites in the leaves were revealed. The increase in the content of phenolic compounds, the total antioxidant activity allowed the plants to survive in adverse environmental conditions. The greatest adaptive potential to drought stress, taking into account the complex of studied physiological and biochemical parameters, was demonstrated by amaranth of cv. Valentina. *A. tricolor* L. cv. Valentina used in the present study can be further investigated as a promising cultivar that can accelerate the breeding for drought tolerance in amaranth.

The leaves of *A. tricolor* L. cv. Valentina contain a sufficient amount of nutraceuticals, phytopigments, and phytochemicals, and the seeds contain a set of macro- and microelements. The leaves of amaranth cv. Valentina can also be used to produce juice as a source of potential nutritional value, phytopigments, antioxidants, flavonoids, phenols, and ascorbic acid in the diet. The present study showed that the cultivars are the sources of biologically active compounds and have an enriched antioxidant profile. The leaves of amaranth A. tricolor cv. Valentina contain a sufficient amount of nutraceuticals, phytopigments, phytochemicals, and the seeds contain a set of macro- and microelements. Valentine's amaranth leaves can also be used to produce juice as a source of potential nutritional value, phytopigments, antioxidants, flavonoids, phenols, and ascorbic acid in the diet. The increased level of the essential macro- and microelements such as Ca, K, P, Mg, Mo, S stipulates the perspective of the functional products creation on the base of the seeds of the studied amaranth (cv. Valentina and Krepysh). The mineral elements concentration in different organs of the plant and their influence on the human life activity are an actual (global) problem, as the deficit of macro- and microelements in the industrial food stuff is extremely huge and dangerous for the human health, because the major part of food stuff is depleted in mineral substances.

The present study showed that the *A. tricolor* L. cv. Valentina and *A. cruentus* L. cv. Krepysh are sources of biologically active compounds and have an enriched antioxidant profile. Recently, the demand for healthy food has increased substantially due to the fact that the link between the health and the consumed products has been shown. In addition to high nutritional value, pseudocereal plants, which include amaranth, contain a large amount of biologically active substances necessary for health. The high protein content of amaranth seeds is characterized by a well-balanced amino acid profile. Seeds are a good source of unsaturated fatty acids, dietary fiber, and essential trace elements. In addition, they contain a wide variety of biologically active compounds. Due to the lack of gluten, these pseudocereals are also interesting ingredients for gluten-free products. Currently, the gluten-free food market is expanding rapidly due to the increasing prevalence of gluten-related diseases such as celiac disease, i.e., gluten intolerance. Amaranth seeds can be used to produce new products, as well as to be an additive to enrich traditional food. Red-colored amaranth leaves can be used to make herbal teas and natural food dyes. The detailed fundamental knowledge of the composition and properties of amaranth seeds is crucial for their introduction into industrial production.

Acknowledgements

The reported study was funded by RFBR and BRFBR, project number 20-516-00012. The reported study was also funded by BRFFR-project number B20R-298.

Conflict of interest

The authors declare no conflict of interest.

Author details

Svetlana Motyleva[1*], Murat Gins[2], Valentina Gins[2], Nikolay Tetyannikov[1], Ivan Kulikov[1], Ludmila Kabashnikova[3], Daria Panischeva[1], Maria Mertvischeva[1] and Irina Domanskaya[3]

1 Federal Horticultural Research Center for Breeding, Agrotechnology and Nursery, Moscow, Russia

2 Federal Research Center of Vegetable Growing, Russia

3 Institute of Biophysics and Cell Engineering of the National Academy of Sciences of Belarus, Belarus

*Address all correspondence to: motyleva_svetlana@mail.ru

References

[1] Hasanuzzaman M, Tanveer M. Handbook of Salt and Drought Stress Tolerance in Plants: Signaling Networks and Adaptive Mechanisms. 1st. ed. Germany: Springer International Publishing; 2020. p. 403. DOI: 10.1007/978-3-030-40277-8

[2] Reddy AR, Chaitanya KV, Vivekanandan M. Mint: Drought-induced responses of photosynthesis and antioxidant metabolism in higher plants. Journal of Plant Physiology. 2004;**161**: 1189-1202. DOI: 10.1016/j.jplph.2004.01.013

[3] Munne-Bosch S, Queval G, Foyer CH. Mint: The impact of global change factors on redox signaling underpinning stress tolerance. Journal of Plant Physiology. 2013;**161**:5-19. DOI: 10.1104/pp.112.205690

[4] Getko NV, Ateslenko EV, Bachishche TS, Kabashnikova LF. Mint: Pigmental leaves foundation of Citrus × *Aurantium* L. in greenhouse culture. Int. Res. J. 2019;**8**(86):57-61. DOI: 10.23670/IRJ.2019.86.8.008

[5] Hernandez JA, Ferrer MA, Jime´nez A, Barcelo´ AR, Sevilla F. Mint: Antioxidant systems and O_2 -/H_2O_2 production in the apoplast of pea leaves. Its relation with salt-induced necrotic lesions in minor veins. Journal of Plant Physiology. 2001;**127**(3):817-831. DOI: 10.1104/pp.010188

[6] Agati G, Tattini M. Mint: Multiple functional roles of flavonoids in photoprotection. The New Phytologist. 2010;**186**(4):786-793. DOI: 10.1111/j.1469-8137.2010.03269.x

[7] Popov AI, Dementyev YN. Mint: Chemical elements of mineral substances in blueberry leaves (Vaccinium uliginosum L.) from the heather family (Ericaceae Juss.). Bulletin of Altai State Agricultural University. 2014;**10**(120): 69-73 (in Russian)

[8] White PJ, Brown PH. Mint: Plant nutrition for sustainable development and global health. Annals of Botany. 2010;**105**(7):1073-1080. DOI: 10.1093/aob/mcq085

[9] Nemtinov V, Kostanchuk Y, Motyleva S, Katskaya A, Timasheva L. Mint: Mineral composition of Allium cepa L. leaves of southern subspecies. Slovak Journal of Food Science. 2020;**14**: 216-223. DOI: 10.5219/1243

[10] Khan KY, Khan MA, Niamat R, Shah GM, Fazal H, Seema N, et al. Mint: Elemental content of some anti-diabetic ethnomedicinal species of genus Ficus Linn. Using atomic absorption spectrophotometry technique. Journal of Medicinal Plants Research. 2012;**6**(11): 2136-2140. DOI: 10.5897/JMPR11.1276

[11] Waraich EA, Ahmad R, Ashraf MY. Mint: Role of mineral nutrition in alleviation of drought stress in plants. Australian Journal of Crop Science. 2011; **5**(6):764-777

[12] Lichtenthaler HK, Bushmann C. Mint: Chlorophylls and carotenoids: Measurement and characterization by UV-VIS spectroscopy. Current Protocols in Food Analytical Chemistry. 2001;**1**(1):F4-3

[13] Velioglu YS, Mazza G, Gao L, Oomah BD. Mint: Antioxidant activity and total phenolics in selected fruits, vegetables, and grain products. Journal of Agricultural and Food Chemistry. 1998; **46**(10):4113-4117. DOI: 10.1021/jf9801973

[14] Brand-Williams W, Cuvelier ME, Berset C. Mint: Use of a free radical

method to evaluate antioxidant activity. Lebensmittel-Wissenschaft und-Technologie. 1995;**28**(1):25-30. DOI: 10.1016/S0023-6438 (95)80008-5

[15] Lebedev AT. Handbook of Mass Spectrometry in Organic Chemistry. Moscow: Tutorial. BINOM. Lab knowledge; 2020. p. 501

[16] Ward D, Olsvig-Whittaker L. Mint: Plant species diversity at the junction of two desert biogeographic zones. Biodiversity Letters. 1993;**1**:172-185

[17] Volk GM, Lynch-Holm VJ, Kostman TA, Goss LJ, Franceschi VR. Mint: The role of druse and raphide calcium oxalate crystals in tissue calcium regulation in Pistia stratiotes leaves. Plant Biology. 2002;**4**(1):34-45. DOI: 10.1055/s-2002-20434

[18] Motyleva SM, Gins MS, Gins VK, Kulikov IM, Kononkov PF, Pivovarov VF, et al. Mint: SEM and EDX analyses for mineral inclusions in the leaves Amaranthus L. AIP Conference Proceedings. 2019;**2068**(1). DOI: 10.1063/1.5089317

[19] Baran EJ, Monje PV. Oxalate biominerals. In: Sigel A, Sigel H, Sigel R, editors. Metal Ions in Life Sciences. Chichester: Wiley; 2008. pp. 219-254

[20] Sanders D, Pellow J, Brownlee C, Herper JF. Mint: Calcium at the crossroads of signaling. The Plant Cell. 2002;**14**:401-417. DOI: 10.1105/tpc.002899

[21] Reddy VS, Reddy AS. Mint: Proteomocs of calcium-signalling components in plants. Phytochemistry. 2004;**65**(12):1745-1776. DOI: 10.1016/j.phytochem.2004.04.033

[22] White PJ. Mint: Calcium signals in root cells: The roles of plasma membrane calcium channels. Biologia. 2004;**59**(S3): 77-83

[23] Poovaiah BW, Reddy ASN, Leopold C. Mint: Calcium messenger system in plants. Critical Reviews in Plant Sciences. 1987;**6**(1):47-103. DOI: 10.1080/07352688709382247

[24] Palta JP. Mint: Stress interactions at the cellular and membrane levels. Horticulture Science. 1990;**25**(11): 1377-1381

[25] Hanson P, Yang RY, Chang LC, Ledesma L, Ledesma D. Mint: Carotenoids, ascorbic acid, minerals, and total glucosinolates in Choysum (B. rapa cv. Parachinensis) and Kailaan (B. oleraceae Alboglabra group) as affected by variety and wet and dry season production. Journal of Food Composition and Analysis. 2011;**24**(7):950-962. DOI: 10.1016/j.jfca.2011.02.001

[26] Kato M, Shimizu S. Mint: Chlorophyll metabolism in higher plants VI. Involvement of peroxidase in chlorophyll degradation. Plant & Cell Physiology. 1985;**26**:1291-1301

[27] Parida AK, Das AB, Sanada Y, Mohanty P. Mint: Effects of salinity on biochemical components of the mangrove Aegiceras corniculatum. Aquatic Botany. 2004;**80**(2):77-87. DOI: 10.1016/j.aquabot.2004.07.005

[28] Jain G, Schwinn KE, Gould KS. Functional role of betalains in Disphyma australe under salinity stress. Environmental and Experimental Botany. 2015;**109**:131-140

[29] Farooq M, Wahid A, Kobayashi N, Fujita D, Basra SMA. Mint: Plant drought stress: Effects, mechanisms and management. Agronomy for Sustainable Development. 2009;**29**:185-212. DOI: 10.1051/agro:2008021

[30] Lin KH, Chao PY, Yang CM, Cheng WC, Lo HF, Chang TR. Mint: The effects of flooding and drought stresses on the antioxidant constituents in sweet potato leaves. Botanical Studies. 2006; **47**(4):417-426

[31] Bettaieb I, Sellami IH, Bourgou S, Limam F, Marzouk B. Mint: Drought effects on polyphenol composition and antioxidant activities in aerial parts of Salvia officinalis L. Acta Physiologiae Plantarum. 2011;**33**(4):1103-1111. DOI: 10.1007/s11738-010-0638-z

[32] Espinoza A, Martina AS, Lopez-Climentb M, Ruiz-Laraa S, Gomez-Cadenasb A, Casarettoa J. Mint: Engineered drought-induced biosynthesis of α-tocopherol alleviates stress-induced leaf damage in tobacco. Journal of Plant Physiology. 2013;**170**(14):1285-1294. DOI: 10.1016/j.jplph.2013.04.004

[33] Bohnert HJ, Jen son RG. Mint: Plant stress adaptations–Making metabolism move. Trends in Biotechnology. 1996;**14**: 267-274. DOI: 10.1016/s1369-5266(98) 80115-5

[34] Lowlor DW. Mint: Limitation to photosynthesis in water stress leaves: Stomata vs. metabolism and the role of ATF. Annals of Botany. 2002;**89**:1-5. DOI: 10.1093/aob/mcf110

[35] Chhetri DR. Mint: Myo-inositol and its derivatives: Their emerging role in the treatment of human diseases. Frontiers in Pharmacology. 2019;**10**:1172. DOI: 10.3389/fphar.2019.01172

[36] Meathnis FG, Ichida AM, Sanders D, Schroeder JI. Mint: Roles of higher plant K+channels. Plant Physiology. 1997; **114**(4):1141-1149. DOI: 10.1104/pp.114.4.1141

[37] Childers D, Corman J, Edwards M, Elser J. Mint: Sustainability challenges of phosphorus and food: Solutions from closing the human phosphorus cycle. Bio Science. 2011;**61**(2):117-124. DOI: 10.1525/bio.2011.61.2.6

[38] Motyleva SM, Kulikov IM, Marchenko LA. Mint: EDS analysis for fruit Prunus elemental composition determination. Material Science Forum. 2017;**888**:314-318. DOI: 10.4028/www.scientific.net/MSF.888.314

[39] Sharifnabia A, Fathibc MH, Eftekhari Yektaa B, Hossainalipouratekhari M. Mint: The structural and bio-corrosion barrier performance of Mg-substituted fluorapatite coating on 316L stainless steel human body implant. Applied Surface Science. 2014;**288**(1):331-340. DOI: 10.1016/j.apsusc.2013.10.029

[40] Schwarz G, Belaidi A. Molybdenum in human health and disease. In: Sigel A, Sigel H, Sigel R, editors. Interrelations between Essential Metal Ions and Human Diseases. Metal Ions in Life Sciences. New York: Springer; 2013. pp. 415-450. DOI: 10.1007/978-94-007-7500-8 13.ch13

[41] Pedersen B, Kalinowski LS, Eggum BO. Mint: The nutritive value of amaranth grain (Amaranthus caudatus L.) protein and minerals of raw and processed grain. Plant Foods for Human Nutrition. 1987;**36**(4):309-324

[42] Avtsyn AP, Zhavoronkov AA, Rishe AA, Strochkova LS. Handbook of Microelementos of Man: Etiology. Classification. Organopathology. Moscow: Medicine; 1991. p. 496 (in Russian)

[43] Nechaev AP, Trauberg SE, Kochetkova AA. Handbook of Food Chemistry. 4th ed. St. Petersburg: Gyord Publishing House; 2007. p. 640 (in Russian)

[44] Vikhreva VA, Khryanin VN, Gins VK, Blinokhvatov AF. Mint: Adaptogenic role of Se in higher plants. Reporter of Bashkirskiy University. Ognostic. 2001;**2**:65-66

[45] Gins MS, Gins VK, Motyleva SM, Kulikov IM, Medvedev SM, Pivovarov VF. Mint: The metabolites of autotrophic and heterotrophic leaves of Amaranthus tricolor L early splendor variety. Agricultural Biology. 2020;**55**(5): 920-931. DOI: 10.15389/agrobiology.2020.5.920eng

[46] Tharun Rao KN, Padhy SK, Dinakaran SK, Banji D, Avasarala H, Ghosh S, Prasad MS. Mint: Pharmacognostic, phytochemical, antimicrobial and antioxidant activity evaluation of *Amaranthus tricolor* Linn. Leaf. Asian Journal of Chemistry. 2012; **24**(1):455-460

[47] Gins MS, Gins VK. Handbook of Food Physiological and Biochemical Basis of Introduction and Selection of Vegetable Cultures. Moscow: PFUR; 2011. p. 190 (in Russian)

[48] Garkaeva TY, Gavrilova OP, Yli-Mattila T, Loskutov IG. Mint: The sources of resistance to *fusarium* head in VIR oat collection. Euphytica. 2013; **191**(3):355-364. DOI: 10.3103/S1068367412010065

[49] Karavaev VA, Gunar LE, Miakin'kov AG, Gins MS, Glazunova SA, Levykina IP, et al. Mint: Slow fluorescence induction and productivity of barley treated with supercritical fluid extract of amaranth. Biofizika. 2012;**57**(4):662-664

[50] Ptushenko V, Gins M, Gins V, Tikhonov A. Mint: Interaction of amaranthin with the electron transport chain of chloroplasts. Russian Journal of Plant Physiology. 2002;**49**:585-591. DOI: 10.102:/A:1020220430690

[51] Amed IM, Cao F, Han Y, Nadira UA, Zhang G, Wu F. Mint: Differential changes in grain ultrastructure, amylase, protein and amino acid profiles between Tibetan wild and cultivated barleys under drought and salinity alone and combined stress. Food Chemistry. 2013; **141**(3):2743-2750. DOI: 10.1016/j.foodchem.2013.05.101

Chapter 9

Review on Pseudo-Cereals of India

Padamnabhi Nagar, Riya Engineer and Krishna Rajput

Abstract

Pseudo-cereals are non-grass, wild plants whose seeds are used in the same manner as cereals, but are underutilized due to the dominance of conventional cereal crops. Pseudo-cereals have varied adaptability. They are climatically more resilient and nutritionally richer than major cereal crops. They are enriched with essential amino acids and their protein content is either similar or greater than that of cereals. They contain adequate amounts of dietary fibers that help improve lipid metabolism. They also contain saponins, polyphenols, betalains, flavonoids, antioxidants, vitamins, and other important phytochemical compounds that help detoxify ROS and cope up with the diseases. Interest in the research of pseudo-cereals is growing among the research community due to its extraordinary nutritional and phytochemical profile and its potential in the development of gluten-free products. It can serve as an alternative food source against staple cereal crops under harsh environmental conditions and if cultivated sustainably, can resolve hunger issues in many countries. Pseudo-cereals form an integral part of the biodiversity due to its widespread usage by the tribals. Wild plants of many angiosperm families are used by tribal communities, but in this review, we will only focus on members of Amaranthceae and Chenopodiaceae families.

Keywords: Amaranthus, quinoa, Amaranthceae, Chenopodiaceae, pseudo-cereals, nutritional profile, gluten-free products

1. Introduction

Majority of the global population in present time is relying heavily on few major cereal crops such as wheat, rice, and maize for nutrition. These handful of crops are sustaining more than 50% of world population. Though they are rich in starch and are consumed for energy needs, they lack some essential micronutrients which has led to hidden hunger among the people. This micronutrient deficiency has affected nearly 2 billion people worldwide and has aroused serious health concerns [1]. This is not only affecting the human health but it also has adverse consequences on other plants such as pseudo-cereals whose biodiversity is declining due to the dominance of conventional cereal crops and for the same reason, they have remained underutilized till date. However, scientists have now turned their attention to the underutilized crops and they are showing considerable interest in pseudo-cereals because of their high resiliency towards the abiotic stress, nutritional, and phytochemical potential and their usage in gluten-free products. In near future, as the human population is predicted to rise, we will need to adopt an interdisciplinary approach to combat food crisis by not only improving the quality of available food by enrichment or biofortification but also by exploring other potential plants which are already enriched with required micronutrients which is an important aspect of food security [2].

Pseudo-cereals that we are going to consider in this review are dicotyledonous plants belonging to families Amaranthceae and Chenopodiaceae for example: *Amaranthus viridis*, *Amaranthus spinosus*, *Achyranthes aspera*, *Celosia aregentea*, and *Chenopodium album*. We will discuss their origin and distribution in brief, their characteristics and how they differ from cereals, their nutritional profiles, and processing techniques that makes them more palatable.

2. A brief of origin and distribution of pseudo-cereals

There are nearly 70 *Amaranthus* species under the family Amaranthceae out of which 17 species produces edible leaves and three species produces grains. *A. viridis* and *A. spinosus* might have originated from south and central America and today they are distributed over tropical and subtropical regions of Africa, South-East Asia, America, and in temperate Europe [3]. *A. aspera* is an herbaceous plant indigenous to Africa and Asia but is now found in nearly 60 tropical and subtropical countries [4]. Genera *Celosia* consists of 60 species all around the world. *C. argentea* is an erect, annual, herbaceous vegetable and is distributed in tropical and subtropical parts of the globe such as South Asia, Africa, and America [5, 6]. *C. album* belonging to the Chenopodiaceae family is an annual plant which is found in wild and is cultivated throughout India. Besides India, it is widely distributed in Europe, North America, Asia, and in different parts of Iran [7].

3. General characters and differences between pseudo-cereals and cereals

The grains of underutilized crops resemble to that of true cereals in functional aspect. However, they differ in nutritional and phytochemical aspects. Pseudo-cereal grains are composed of less of starch and more of proteins and lipids as opposed to cereals. The reason is, anatomically, pseudo-cereal grain contains lesser amount of endosperm (starch storing organ) and greater amount of embryo (that store proteins and lipids). Pseudo-cereals possess a considerable amount of essential amino acids such as lysine, cysteine, and methionine. Other than lysine, *Amaranthus* comprises of an adequate quantity of arginine and histidine which are inevitable nutrients for new born and children. Proteins in pseudo-cereals and cereals differ in their storage forms. In cereals, proteins are stored in the form of prolamins whereas in pseudo-cereals proteins are present in the form of globulins and albumins. High concentration of prolamins in cereals is responsible for disease like celiac disease. Therefore, pseudo-cereals are being sought out as an alternative to cereals for gluten-free diet. Studies have shown that dietary fibers found in *Amaranthus* are approximately in the same range as that of wheat. Regarding vitamins and minerals, the value of thiamine content has been found to be greater in amaranth than in wheat. Riboflavin, vitamin-C, folic acid, and vitamin-E are also prominent in amaranth. It has been observed that gluten-free products and ultimately gluten-free diets are deficient in calcium, magnesium, and iron. Thus, richer calcium content in pseudo-cereals is relevant for the people suffering from celiac disease, osteopenia, and osteoporosis. Fats in pseudo-cereals are more than in cereals especially high unsaturated fatty acids (particularly linolenic acid) are characteristic of pseudo-cereals. Amaranthus contains "squalene" which is a highly unsaturated, open chain triterpene which is exclusively found in the liver of deep-sea fish and other marine species. Lipid content is two to three times higher in pseudo-cereals than in cereals. This highly unsaturated lipids are also stable against oxidation which is a desirable trait. This feature is accredited to the tocopherols existing in relatively higher amounts [8]. In cereal grains, there are some anti-nutrients such as phytate, tannins, and saponins that interfere with nutrient absorption and utilization which are found in comparatively lesser quantities in pseudo-cereals. Hence, their nutrient profile makes them a suitable candidate for gluten-free products and are therefore in high demand among the consumers around the world, mainly among the celiac disease patients. This high caloric content and balanced amino acids in pseudo-cereals are advantageous to cope up with micronutrient deficiency in developing and under-developed countries [9].

A. viridis and *A. spinosus* are an excellent source of protein with lysine and methionine and phytochemicals such as carotenoids, ascorbic acid, dietary fibers, and minerals such as Ca, Mg, K, P, Fe, Zn, Cu, and Mn. They are an impressive source of antioxidants and vitamins which is why they have great importance in food industry. They are consumed as cooked, steamed, or fried vegetables [3].

A. aspera is an important source of biologically active trace elements and metals. It is rich in Fe, Cu, Ca, and Na [10]. Leaves of *A. aspera* predominantly comprises of fats, saponins, flavonoids, alkaloids, and tannins. These phytochemicals, especially phenolic compounds are responsible for the harmful ROS scavenging property of the plant that makes it a potential source of human nutrition [11].

In the extracts of *Celosia argentea*, the characteristic phyto-constituents determined were cyclic peptides, phenols, saponins, amino acids, flavonoids, alkaloids, and tannins. Saponins among all are the principal pharmacologically active agents but are needed to be explored further for their bioactivity and usefulness. Apart from saponins, higher concentration of fats renders the plant eligible as an energetic and nutritional candidate for mal-nourished children [12, 13].

The determination of vitamin-C and β-carotene from the young as well as mature shoots of *C. album* indicated that it can serve as an interesting supplement of vitamins in the diet bowl. Also, there were prominent amounts of nutrients such as proteins, crude alkaloids, and saponins along with elements like potassium, calcium, zinc, and iron but on the contrary, dietary fibers were little less. All the above-mentioned components have beneficial impact on our health [14].

4. Nutritional profile

This section deals with the nutritional aspect of chosen *A. viridis*, *A. aspera*, and *C. album* in context of their protein, carbohydrate, fat, dietary fiber, and vitamin and mineral composition. Nutritional composition of major cereals, that is, wheat, rice, and maize are incorporated for comparative study (**Tables 1**–7).

4.1 *A. viridis*

Nutrients	Concentration (g/100 g)
Protein	14.95 ± 0.19^{c}
Fat	6.30 ± 0.05^{a}
Total sugars	0.27 ± 0.01^{b}
Soluble fiber	0.68 ± 0.01^{c}
Insoluble fiber	29.92 ± 0.01^{d}
Carbohydrates	28.55 ± 0.76^{a}
Essential minerals	(mg/g)
Calcium (Ca)	5.97 ± 0.27^{d}
Potassium (K)	6.66 ± 0.19^{c}
Magnesium (Mg)	4.27 ± 0.02^{d}
Sodium (Na)	0.77 ± 0.01^{d}
Phosphorous (P)	8.73 ± 0.02^{a}
Trace elements	
Iron (Fe) (mg/g)	0.33 ± 0.23^{a}
Chromium (Cr) (µg/g)	5.36 ± 0.01^{b}
Copper (Cu) (µg/g)	6.14 ± 0.01^{b}
Zinc (Zn) (µg/g)	24.95 ± 0.01^{b}

Average followed by different letters on the same line indicate statistical difference according to the Duncan test ($p \leq 0.05$).

Table 1.
Chemical composition of Amaranthus viridis (grains) in dry basis [15].

4.2 *A. aspera*

Nutrients	Concentration (g/100 g)
Crude protein	36.71
Crude fat	8.31
Carbohydrates	37.52
Crude fiber	0.44

Table 2.
Proximate chemical composition of Achyranthes aspera (seeds) in dry basis [16].

Minerals	Concentration
Macro-minerals	(mg/g)
Sodium (Na)	0.06 ± 0.01^{b}
Potassium (K)	6.35 ± 0.04^{b}
Calcium (Ca)	0.17 ± 0.01^{b}
Magnesium (Mg)	2.18 ± 0.01^{b}
Trace minerals	(µg/g)
Molybdenum (Mo)	0.28 ± 0.02^{b}
Manganese (Mn)	30.20 ± 0.63^{b}
Aluminum (Al)	41.07 ± 4.16^{b}

Minerals	Concentration
Iron (Fe)	76.82 ± 4.15^b
Zinc (Zn)	41.77 ± 0.18^a
Copper (Cu)	7.67 ± 0.19^b
Strontium (Sr)	3.39 ± 0.26^b
Cadmium (Cd)	0.10 ± 0.04^b
Lead (Pb)	0.21 ± 0.02^b
Ultra-trace minerals	(μg/g)
Chromium (Cr)	2.18 ± 0.38^b
Cobalt (Co)	0.09 ± 0.01^b
Nickel (Ni)	1.35 ± 0.44^b
Tin (Sn)	0.18 ± 0.04^b

Means (±SEM) sharing different letters in the same row are significantly ($P < 0.05$) different ($n = 3$).

Table 3.
Mineral composition of Achyranthes aspera seeds (dry powder) [17].

4.3 *C. album*

Nutrients	Concentration (g/100 g)
Protein	13.12^b ± 0.07
Fat	6.50^a ± 0.30
Crude fiber	13.09^b ± 0.04
Carbohydrate	54.61^a ± 0.09
Total starch	41.44^a ± 0.29

Mean values in the same row which is not followed by the same letter are significantly different ($p < 0.05$). Values represent mean ± standard deviation ($n = 3$).

Table 4.
Proximate composition of Chenopodium album (flour) [18].

Minerals	Concentration (mg/kg)
Calcium (Ca)	177.89^a ± 4.04
Sodium (Na)	82.45^b ± 0.42
Iron (Fe)	112.07^a ± 1.26
Magnesium (Mg)	1600.34^a ± 15.01
Copper (Cu)	5.90^b ± 0.36
Zinc (Zn)	24.20^b ± 0.23
Potassium (K)	10113.31^a ± 21.50

Mean values in the same row which is not followed by the same letter are significantly different ($p \leq 0.05$). Values represent mean ± standard deviation ($n = 3$).

Table 5.
Mineral composition of Chenopodium album (flour) [19].

4.4 *Zea mays* (maize), *Triticum aestivum* (wheat), and *Oryza sativa* (rice)

Cereals	Protein	Fat	Fiber	Carbohydrate
Wheat	12.39 ± 0.010	2.50 ± 0.010	1.14 ± 0.070	75.65 ± 0.240
Maize	8.58 ± 0.000	2.85 ± 0.020	2.83 ± 0.020	75.39 ± 0.030
Rice	10.49 ± 0.010	3.94 ± 0.030	1.09 ± 0.000	75.61 ± 0.450

Values reported were average of duplicate analysis.

Table 6.
Proximate composition (%) of cereals [20].

Cereals	Wheat	Maize	Rice
Sodium (Na)	383.33 ± 0.001	333.33 ± 0.0011	126.67 ± 0.001
Potassium (K)	416.67 ± 0.001	300.00 ± 0.001	183.33 ± 0.001
Calcium (Ca)	60.02 ± 0.0027	12.95 ± 0.7770	3.35 ± 0.0019
Magnesium (Mg)	140.73 ± 0.0053	77.62 ± 0.0037	23.67 ± 0.0052
Iron (Fe)	67.22 ± 0.0011	58.35 ± 0.0006	59.33 ± 0.0005
Zinc (Zn)	11.73 ± 0.0011	9.45 ± 0.0009	9.27 ± 0.0006

Mean ± standard deviation.

Table 7.
Mineral composition (mg/100 g) of cereals [20].

5. Processing treatments for pseudo-cereals

Their extraordinary nutritional profile is the result of the presence of countless bioactive components that includes essential amino acids, proteins, phenolic compounds, and a wide range of anti-oxidants, thus rendering them with a high nutraceutical potential. But along with favorable substances, they also contain anti-nutrients such as phytate, tannins, and saponins which reduces the bioavailability of beneficial supplements. To resolve this, pseudo-cereals are subjected to several processing treatments like soaking, fermentation, popping, germination, and cooking. Such treatments improve bioavailability of nutrients by decreasing the amount of anti-nutrients and consequently enhances the nutritional value of pseudo-cereals. For example, seeds of *Amaranthus* are consumed as popped, sprouted, baked, or grounded into flour and cooked as porridge [21].

5.1 Processing treatments

Processing increases the digestibility and palatability of respective food product. It extends the self-life and reduces the anti-nutritional compounds. Following are few traditional methods for processing pseudo-cereals to make them more consumable.

5.1.1 Fermentation

Fermentation is a metabolic process carried out by anaerobic microorganisms in which carbohydrates are broken down to release energy. It is an age-old technique for food preservation. Pseudo-cereals are an adequate source of carbohydrates, minerals, vitamins, sterols, and other growth factors that sustains the microbe populations.

These grains are composed of an indigenous microbiota comprising of molds, lactic acid bacteria (LAB), enterobacteria, etc. LAB are gram positive, strictly fermentative bacteria which carries out lactic acid fermentation and produces lactic acid as the major metabolic end product of carbohydrate fermentation and the most frequently used strain for this purpose is *Lactobacillus plantarum*.

Lactic acid fermentation is a commonly used food processing technique which can be employed in many different ways to improve nutritional and functional quality of pseudo-cereals such as production of bioactive peptides to stimulate immune system, increasing total phenolic content and antioxidant capacity, decreasing of anti-nutritional factors like phytic acid, tannins, and enzyme inhibitors. The formation of lactic acid during fermentation leads to a decrease in pH that results in enhanced activity of endogenous phytase. Phytases constitutes particular subgroup of phosphatases which are responsible for lowering or eliminating the anti-nutritional effect of phytic acid. Some LAB strains and other vitamin producing microorganisms can elevate the concentrations of natural form of vitamins that leads to the decrease in side effects of chemically synthesized vitamins. Hence, they can be utilized as an alternative source of biofortification which is also a cost-effective strategy and eliminates the need to add synthetic vitamins. Food products consumed after fermentation with LAB improves the overall nutritional quality by increasing vitamin B9 concentrations. There is a need to explore more beneficial effects of lactic acid fermentation to design novel and healthier edibles especially for patients with celiac disease [22, 23].

5.1.2 Popping

Also known as heat induced puffing, is a low-cost technology in which heating at atmospheric pressure gives rise to high internal pressure due to evaporation of moisture, causing the pericarp to break, leading to the expansion of endosperm. Puffed grains undergo dehydration as well as structural and textural changes. Puffing increases digestibility and functionality of the grains. Because of such modifications, *Amaranthus* flour has been proposed to be used as an ingredient in bakery products. Puffed grains are ready-to-eat products, also incorporated in the snack formulations [24].

5.1.3 Germination

Germination is a process in which a new plant arises from the seed if the seed is under favorable conditions. Imbibition is the first step in germination process in which the dry seed absorbs water which leads to the increased metabolic rates and subsequent growth. The interesting part is the rise of hydrolytic enzyme activities followed by breakdown of stored macromolecules in the seed. Such changes alter the technological properties and functionality of grains which is a desirable asset. During germination, the action of hydrolytic enzymes on starch increases its digestibility. It also increases the content of free amino acids which are readily absorbed compared to the intact proteins, influencing the postprandial protein metabolism. The breakdown of cell wall changes the solubility of fiber components and increases the amounts of bioactive compounds and antioxidant activities [25].

5.1.4 Cooking

Grains of pseudo-cereals are generally eaten after boiling. However, excessive boiling decreases the phenolic contents of the grains. Highest retention of phenolic contents was observed by pressure cooking. From anti-nutritional aspect, no significant reduction was seen in anti-nutritional compounds, especially of phytic acid through boiling. Evaluation of minerals in *Amaranthus* revealed that boiling and steaming negatively affected the folate content and also certain essential amino acids [26].

6. Conclusion

Pseudo-cereals are a powerhouse of nutrients. There is a need to explore them further and bring them in our daily diet. Even though pseudo-cereals seem more superior than cereals in context of their chemical composition, the anti-nutrients present in them reduces the bioavailability of the nutritional components. Phytate and lower inositol phosphates binds to the minerals like calcium, zinc, magnesium, and iron, making them unavailable for absorption [26]. As nutritional deficiency is becoming more prevalent among the human population throughout the globe, food producers are expected to develop novel strategies for their improved processing. Moreover, there is a requirement of making people aware about the benefits of pseudo-cereals so that they consider them in their diet along with the cereals which will also elevate the nutritional quality of their diet. Prerequisite for this is to design new range of food products prepared using pseudo-cereals as their key ingredients and introduce them into the market. Pseudo-cereals are also in demand for the manufacture of gluten-free edibles. Therefore, it is very important to have a detailed understanding of the properties of pseudo-cereals and their benefits and drawbacks. This will aid in boosting the quality of life of the people with celiac and other gluten-induced diseases. Pseudo-cereals have an immeasurable potential, the only task is to give an eye to them.

Acknowledgements

Thanks to the head of the Department of Botany, Faculty of Science, The Maharaja Sayajirao University of Baroda for providing laboratory facilities at the department.

Author details

Padamnabhi Nagar*, Riya Engineer and Krishna Rajput
The Maharaja Sayajirao University of Baroda, Vadodara, India

*Address all correspondence to: padamnabhi.nagar-botany@msubaroda.ac.in

References

[1] FAO. The State of Food and Agriculture. Rome: Food and Agriculture Organization; 2013

[2] Pirzadah TB, Malik B. Pseudocereals as super foods of 21st century: Recent technological interventions. Journal of Agriculture and Food Research. 2020;**2**:100052

[3] Sarker U, Oba S. Nutraceuticals, antioxidant pigments, and phytochemicals in the leaves of *Amaranthus spinosus* and *Amaranthus viridis* weedy species. Scientific Reports. 2019;**9**(1):20413

[4] Holm L, Doll J, Holm E, Pancho JV, Herberger JP. World Weeds: Natural Histories and Distribution. United States: John Wiley & Sons; 1997

[5] Ayodele JT, Olajide OS. Proximate and amino acid composition of *Celosia argentea* leaves. Nigerian Journal of Basic and Applied Sciences. 2011;**19**(1):162-165

[6] Feng N, Xue Q, Guo Q, Zhao R, Guo M. Genetic diversity and population structure of *Celosia argentea* and related species revealed by SRAP. Biochemical Genetics. 2009;**47**(7):521-532

[7] Jan R, Saxena DC, Singh S. Effect of germination on nutritional, functional, pasting, and microstructural properties of chenopodium (*Chenopodium album*) flour. Journal of Food Processing and Preservation. 2017;**41**(3):e12959

[8] Mir NA, Riar CS, Singh S. Nutritional constituents of pseudo cereals and their potential use in food systems: A review. Trends in Food Science & Technology. 2018;**75**:170-180

[9] Bekkering CS, Tian L. Thinking outside of the cereal box: Breeding underutilized (pseudo) cereals for improved human nutrition. Frontiers in Genetics. 2019;**10**:1289

[10] Fatima N, Dar NG, Imran H, Sohail T, Asghar U, Yaqeen Z, et al. Evaluation of nutritional and sub-acute toxicological study of plant based supplement of *Achyranthes aspera*. Pakistan Journal of Pharmaceutical Sciences. 2014;**27**(5):1199-1202

[11] Priya CL, Kumar G, Karthik L, Rao KB. Phytochemical composition and in vitro antioxidant activity of *Achyranthes aspera* Linn (Amaranthaceae) leaf extracts. Journal of Agricultural Technology. 2012;**8**(1):143-156

[12] Fayaz M, Bhat MH, Kumar A, Jain AK. Phytochemical screening and nutritional analysis of some parts of *Celosia argentea* L. Chemical Science. 2019;**8**(1):12-19

[13] Tang Y, Xin HL, Guo ML. Review on research of the phytochemistry and pharmacological activities of *Celosia argentea*. Revista Brasileira de Farmacognosia. 2016;**26**:787-796

[14] Pandey S, Gupta RK. Screening of nutritional, phytochemical, antioxidant and antibacterial activity of *Chenopodium album* (Bathua). Journal of Pharmacognosy and Phytochemistry. 2014;**3**(3):1-9

[15] Silva AD, Ávila S, Küster RT, Dos Santos MP, Grassi MT, de Queiroz Pereira Pinto C, et al. In vitro bioaccessibility of proteins, phenolics, flavonoids and antioxidant activity of *Amaranthus viridis*. Plant Foods for Human Nutrition. 2021;**76**(4):478-486

[16] Kumar N, Sharma J, Singh SP, Singh A, Krishna VH, Chakrabarti R. Validation of

growth enhancing, immunostimulatory and disease resistance properties of *Achyranthes aspera* in *Labeo rohita* fry in pond conditions. Heliyon. 2019; **5**(2):e01246

[17] Kumar NE, Sharma JA, Kumar G, Shrivastav AK, Tiwari NE, Begum AJ, et al. Evaluation of nutritional value of prickly chaff flower (*Achyranthes aspera*) as fish feed ingredient. The Indian Journal of Animal Sciences. 2021;**91**(3):239-244

[18] Jan R, Saxena DC, Singh S. Physico-chemical, textural, sensory and antioxidant characteristics of gluten-free cookies made from raw and germinated Chenopodium (*Chenopodium album*) flour. LWT- Food Science and Technology. 2016;**71**:281-287

[19] Jan R, Saxena DC, Singh S. Comparative study of raw and germinated Chenopodium (*Chenopodium album*) flour on the basis of thermal, rheological, minerals, fatty acid profile and phytocomponents. Food Chemistry. 2018;**269**:173-180

[20] Abdulrahman WF, Omoniyi AO. Proximate analysis and mineral compositions of different cereals available in Gwagwalada market, FCT, Abuja, Nigeria. Advance Journal of Food Science and Technology. 2016;**3**(2):50-55

[21] Thakur P, Kumar K. Nutritional importance and processing aspects of pseudo-cereals. Journal of Agricultural Engineering and Food Technology. 2019;**6**:155-160

[22] Castro-Alba V, Lazarte CE, Perez-Rea D, Carlsson NG, Almgren A, Bergenståhl B, et al. Fermentation of pseudocereals quinoa, canihua, and amaranth to improve mineral accessibility through degradation of phytate. Journal of the Science of Food and Agriculture. 2019;**99**(11):5239-5248

[23] Rollán GC, Gerez CL, LeBlanc JG. Lactic fermentation as a strategy to improve the nutritional and functional values of pseudocereals. Frontiers in Nutrition. 2019;**6**:98

[24] Paucar-Menacho LM, Dueñas M, Peñas E, Frias J, Martínez-Villaluenga C. Effect of dry heat puffing on nutritional composition, fatty acid, amino acid and phenolic profiles of pseudocereals grains. Polish Journal of Food and Nutrition Sciences. 2018;**68**(4)

[25] Mäkinen OE, Arendt EK. Nonbrewing applications of malted cereals, pseudocereals, and legumes: A review. Journal of the American Society of Brewing Chemists. 2015;**73**(3):223-227

[26] Henrion M, Labat E, Lamothe L. Pseudocereals as healthy grains: An overview. In: Innovative Processing Technologies for Healthy Grains. United States: John Wiley & Sons Ltd.; 2021. pp. 37-59